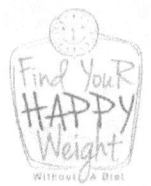

Find Your Happy Weight
Without A Diet

The Neuroscience of Weight Loss

Dr Peter Steidl

If your weight is causing you a serious health problem or risk, then this book is not for you. You need to see a medical expert and accept their guidance.

If you are pregnant, I ask you to defer reading this book until your pregnancy is over. You need to consider the nutritional requirements of your unborn child and your medical practitioner is the best source of information for this.

I have written this book for the tens of millions of people around the world who are trying to lose weight, typically by going on a diet, for lifestyle and general health reasons. They tend to struggle with the deprivation a diet brings, lose some weight and then put it back on again. For the vast majority of people, diets don't work. In fact, diets are making them less healthy!

Should you be neither battling with health problems nor going through a pregnancy but are one of the tens of millions of people who are not happy with their weight then I invite you to read on.... In this book, I will explain not only why dieting is a health hazard but also why diets typically don't work, and, most importantly, what you can do to reach your Happy Weight – and this does not involve dieting!

Contents

About you – and the book you are about to read

Given that you are holding my book in your hands, it would make sense to go through a little introduction. Have a look at the statements below and tick (literally or in your mind) all those that apply to you:

☐ I am overweight and want to lose weight

☐ When I go on a diet, I tend to give up before I have lost the weight I set out to lose.

☐ When I go on a diet, I lose weight but then put it back on again.

☐ When I want to lose weight, I make a detailed plan – how much weight to lose, by when, what I will be allowed to eat, and so forth. I follow my plan for a while but then I fall back into my old eating habits.

☐ I have tried a commercial weight loss program but it didn't work for me.

☐ I am under a lot of stress, and when I'm stressed I tend to fall back into my old eating habits.

☐ I typically stick with my weight loss program for most of the time, but when I get tired in the evening I just binge eat.

☐ There is already so much change around me – in my work, my family life, or with my friends or financial situation – that on top of all this I find it hard to concentrate on losing weight.

☐ I commit to losing weight, and then, one day, I realize I have gone back to many of my old eating habits.

☐ I have tried and failed so often before when trying to lose weight that I have stopped expecting to succeed.

The more statements you have ticked, the more useful this book will be to you. If you haven't ticked any, you may still gain something from reading this book, or perhaps you can use the book as a Christmas present for somebody who is likely to tick some of these boxes?

Clearly, I don't know you personally, but I do know what happens with the majority of people who want to lose weight, and there is a fair chance that much of what I have learned about them applies to you as well. Many of these Weight Warriors have used several diets over the years, and they have found that they either don't stick with a diet for long enough to reach their goal weight, or they lose the weight and then put it on again when they finish their diet. And most of them even put on a bit more.

The number of overweight people is increasing every year. In developed countries, this has been happening for many years, and more recently developing countries have started to show the same trend.

So what are the conclusions we can draw from this?

First, and most importantly, you can be absolutely certain that you are not alone in your quest! There are literally hundreds of millions of people around the world who want to lose weight. You are one of a huge army of Weight Warriors.

Second, few people seem to have worked out how to lose weight successfully. Given that there are a multitude of free diets as well as commercial weight-loss programs, and plenty of people who will try anything to make their weight loss happen, we surely could have expected a *decrease* in the number of overweight people. But we have seen exactly the opposite.

The only reasonable conclusion is that the approach typically used to losing weight isn't working.

I am not suggesting that nobody has ever lost weight on a diet and then been able to maintain their weight afterward. Obviously, there are exceptions, but my point is that these are *exceptions* rather than the rule. If you find it difficult to lose weight, you are part of the dominant majority of people.

Why then another book on weight loss? Is there a 'new' way to lose weight that promises much better results?

There is, because neuroscience research is teaching us why it is so difficult for you to lose weight. Neuroscience is a branch of medical science that focuses on how the human brain works. Much progress has been made in our understanding of why we do what we do, mainly through diagnostic technologies that allow us to observe what is happening in the brain.

This has led to an important realization: for decades, we have been focusing on the wrong issue. The focus of many weight programs and diets is on eating less and eating different foods. As counterintuitive as it may sound, this is the main reason why these programs show such a low success rate.

As long as you keep going on a diet to lose weight and try your hardest to follow this diet, you are not likely to succeed. The proof can be seen in the hundreds of millions of people who have done just that and failed.

This takes me to the content of the book you are holding in your hands.

What I am presenting to you is a very different approach to losing weight. It is based on research in the fields of neuroscience and psychology. Don't fear; this is not about simply visualizing that you can lose weight and then waking up one day finding you have lost it. I am not into esoteric methods, nor do I believe in the 'magnetism' of thought. If weight loss were that easy, we wouldn't have hundreds of millions of people fighting such a frustrating battle.

I don't want to give it all away in the first few pages, but let me very briefly outline where this book will take you:

First I will explain some fundamental issues: the fact that you – like the vast majority of people – are designed *to put on weight*. Yes, you read that correctly: your brain, just like the brain of anyone else, is designed to make you eat and to avoid losing weight. It is natural to overeat. But unfortunately it is neither useful nor healthy.

Second, I will help you to understand why diets don't work. Millions of people around the world go on diets that don't deliver. Many of them don't even expect the diet to do so, but for them it's like buying a lottery ticket: you don't expect to win, but you buy it anyway just in case you happen to get lucky. The problem with diets is not just that they don't work; there is evidence to show that diets actually cause you to *put on* more weight once you have finished with them. I will explain why this happens in some detail, because it is important to understand the impact diets have on your eating behavior.

Third, I will help you gain an understanding of how your mind works when it comes to losing weight. I won't use medical terms or go through in-depth scientific explanations. Rather, I will present you with insights into what is happening in your mind when you try to lose weight.

I will then offer you a very different approach to reaching and maintaining your Happy Weight. This approach focuses on what is driving you to eat (your Eating Drivers) and what is making it difficult for you to change your eating behavior and holding you back (the Barriers).

If you can effectively deal with the Eating Drivers and the Barriers, you will not only lose weight but be able to maintain your new weight once the excess is gone. Clearly, we have to talk about food as well, but let me assure you food should not be the focus of your efforts. At least, not until you have made progress in dealing with your Eating Drivers and Barriers.

In order to lose weight successfully, you will need something that seems to be in short supply these days: patience.

Research has shown that serial dieters start a new diet every 18 months on average. That seems to be the time it takes them to finish their last diet, realize that it didn't work, get over their disappointment and get ready to try something else.

These serial dieters typically fail in their efforts. They have shown us that there is no point in going from diet to diet and setting unrealistic goals only to fail in the end and possibly put on even more weight. Wouldn't it be better to give yourself the time you need to address your weight issues once and for all? What if it takes you six or nine months? Or even a year? Finding a solution to your weight problem that lasts you for the rest of your life must surely be better than becoming (or staying) a serial dieter!

Back to the Happy Weight book.

When making use of this book, you could simply go to the action part, develop your very own tailor-made action program and start making progress. However, I encourage you *not* to do this. It is important that you understand why it is so difficult to lose weight. Naturally, action is all important, but you will find that you will make much better progress if you know what you have to achieve and why.

The first part aims to help you build a solid foundation of knowledge and develop an understanding of the eating drivers and barriers you must address to be successful. It proposes that you take a measured approach by focusing on weight maintenance rather than on weight loss. The recommended actions are designed to deal with the most basic yet very important issues that tend to hold many Weight Warriors back.

The second part deals with some of the massive drivers and barriers many people experience. More specifically, I present strategies for changing bad eating habits and for creating good ones. As you will require a measure of willpower to do this, I also cover the depletion and development of willpower. I deal with the topic of stress and offer you practical advice on actions you can take to more effectively manage stress or even eliminate it from your life.

Finally, there is an important point I must stress again: *If you are battling health problems or experiencing a pregnancy, then this book is not for you. You need to rely on your doctor to develop a tailor-made program for you.* I have written this book for the many dieters who try to lose weight yet don't succeed, who may be worried about their health but are (not yet) battling serious health problems, and who are sick and tired of being on a diet treadmill and want to put a life-long solution in place.

If this includes you, then I sincerely hope you will find the content of this book useful and that you will act on it. This will allow you to not only shed weight but to reach and maintain your Happy Weight without struggle or sacrifice. After all, the goal we all share is to have a happy, healthier life. Finding our Happy Weight can make a solid contribution to that!

Dr Peter Steidl
October 2012

Send me an email if you have any questions or comments or simply want to be kept informed about future Happy Weight publications or activities.

*My email address is **peter@petersteidl.com***

PART I
The Foundation

1

You are designed to eat – a lot!

Your brain is designed to encourage you to eat. Your stress response is designed to help you put on weight. Your ability to habitualize has created some bad eating habits.

These are some of the odds you are up against! Anyone who attempts to lose weight and maintain their lower weight is bound to struggle, unless they understand the forces that drive them to eat and learn how to eliminate or at least weaken these forces.

In the following chapters, I explore these forces in greater depth. In Part II, I present ways of eliminating or at least weakening these forces, allowing you to lose weight in a healthy, sensible way and, most importantly, to maintain the lower weight once you have reached it!

Eric's story

Eric opens his eyes, surprised and relieved. It is dark. For a moment he thinks he is on a train. The he realizes the sound is coming from the guy next to him. Such a snore! That's probably what woke him up. He remembers that the guy – was it Fred? – hasn't had his surgery yet; it had to be delayed because he's carrying too much weight.

At any other time, Eric might have been annoyed by the pain in his chest or the snoring of his roommate. But not today. He's happy to be there and to be alive, even though the pain isn't the most appealing way to prove this to himself.

Memories start flooding back. It was only a few weeks ago, but now it seems like months, an eternity in fact, that he went to see his GP to complain about being short of breath and feeling dizzy when walking even just a short distance.

On top of that, he had been feeling really down, lacking in energy and unable to concentrate. And none of this was exactly helping either his marriage or his work. He was only in his early fifties, for crying out loud – surely this couldn't be an age-related thing? Sure, he was overweight – maybe a bit obese if he was honest about it.

Can you be a bit obese? he had wondered. *Anyway, everyone has his vices. Some smoke, some drink, some gamble, some take drugs; I just eat... and, well, maybe drink a bit. How bad can that be?*

The GP had nodded his head wisely and referred Eric to a cardiologist.

'It's your heart!' the cardiologist had cheerfully announced. 'We have to get it fixed or you could be dead within the year! I wouldn't start listening to Wagner's complete *Ring* or reading the Larsen trilogy if I were you – you might never find out what happens at the end....' He chuckled. He clearly thought he was hilarious. But Eric couldn't see the funny side to it. Not then, and not now.

But something must have happened, because as he listened to the cardiologist his dizziness disappeared. It was replaced by an absolute clarity of mind and a hollow feeling in the center of his body. It felt like he had a big hole in there, hollow and empty. And a clear thought emerged in his mind: *I am going to die!*

I shouldn't have eaten all this crap food! he thought ruefully on the way home from the hospital, *or at least not so much of it....*

Remorse set in.

If I get through this, he promised himself, *I will change. I will eat healthy food, lose weight and stay on the straight and narrow!* And in his damaged heart, he knew that before all this was over, he would have offered God a deal: *Let me live and I will change!*

By the time he ends up at the cardiothoracic surgeon's office – the guy who will eventually use a band saw to cut Eric's chest open, reach into the cavity and, hopefully, fix the problem – he is resigned to his fate. Fear has morphed into depression. He spends sleepless nights thinking about all the things he had planned to do but now may not be able to do after all, and all the loose ends he may never be able to tie up....

He puts on a brave face for the world, but inside the waiting and uncertainty is tearing him up. *Better to get this over and done with – whichever way it goes – than to just wait for something to happen*, he concludes.

Then the big day comes.

He remembers checking into his hospital room, getting prepped the next morning and then, already pretty much out of it, being wheeled into the operating theatre for the anesthetic.

He re-lives the surprise he felt when he first woke up. There would have been elation, had it not been for the huge plastic thing they had stuck down his throat to help him breathe. Just focusing on taking his next breath, and the one after that, was all he could cope with, until the recovery ward nurse finally decided he was out of danger and eased his suffering a bit by removing the annoying contraption.

From then on, pain was Eric's constant partner in this enterprise, but the surgeon told him it had all gone smoothly and that he should recover fully, so that, Eric thinks, is worth feeling a bit of pain for!

After a day or so, a hospital dietician visits him. She tells him he brought all this on himself by eating so much rubbish. *No point arguing*, Eric thinks. *She's seen the food questionnaire I filled out when I was admitted; she knows how much junk I've been eating....*

Eric doesn't mind being reprimanded by the dietician. In fact, he's grateful. This is a new start. What he did in the past lies in the past. From now on, his life will be different.

Until he is discharged, the dietician visits Eric every day to discuss his personalized diet solution and give him pamphlets to read. She points out how he might be able to relax his diet a bit over time but warns him about falling back into his old eating habits. *As if I ever would*, Eric thinks, *given what I've just been through!*

Linda's Story

Linda is the Chief Dietician at a major metropolitan hospital, and her special responsibility is heart surgery patients with weight problems. She takes her role seriously and believes that a good diet and a bit of exercise can help patients recover more quickly.

Heart patients have a special place in her mind. Obesity, eating bad food and limiting exercise to walking from the couch to the fridge and back again are major contributors to the health issues that have brought many of the patients she sees to the hospital. Linda, whose work has been recognized by her peers, is determined to make a difference.

When Linda is invited to speak at a national conference, she decides to follow up with some of the past heart patients who she helped during their recovery by teaching them about the importance of a healthy diet.

The idea is to turn up unexpectedly to see her patients, thus avoiding the situation where patients who want to be seen as doing the right thing may misrepresent their eating habits rather than be completely honest.

The first patient on her list is Eric. She remembers him well; he was devastated by his heart surgery. Heart surgery is a major, life-changing event for many, but Eric was one of those intense patients who really, really wanted to know what to do to avoid ending up in hospital again. He was a star pupil, drinking it all in. He should make a pretty good case study for the conference, she thought.

She arrives at his address and rings the bell. When the door opens, she recognizes Eric, who looks more stunned than surprised. Maybe he's just happy to see her. Fortuitously, he is having his afternoon tea. Can she join him, Linda asks. He is reluctant, but what can he do? He invites Linda in.

'What are you having?' she asks politely. Then she wishes she hadn't asked. She wishes Eric was not on the randomly selected list of patients to be followed up. She wishes she never had this silly idea of going to people's homes to check up on them. She wishes she had never received the invitation to present a paper at the conference. Greasy fish and chips for afternoon tea!

She goes through the routine and checks the fridge: ice cream, mayonnaise, chocolate, some chemical goo masquerading as a pudding, leftover pizza, and... on goes the long list of horrors. The pantry isn't any better.

When confronted with this evidence, Eric admits that it didn't take him very long to fall back into his old habits.

'When I started to feel really great again', he explains, 'I thought I could reward myself a bit for what I had been through. Just a bit of something I really like eating. But it was a bit more of the old stuff every day, until one day I realized I'd gone right back to where I was before all this started.'

'But I feel great', he tries to reason. 'I really feel much better than I've felt for years! And I'm working on improving my diet.'

There is no evidence of that really, Linda thinks, but to change this guy you'd have to force feed him the right food. He isn't going to make it. What a waste....

Footnote: A major metropolitan hospital that provided an extensive education service for heart surgery patients followed up a sample of past patients. The objective was to assess the impact of providing dietary advice to heart surgery patients during recovery where diet had been a likely contributor to their heart disease.

The findings showed that the majority of patients went back to the same unhealthy diets that contributed to their heart problems in the first place.

On the face of it, you'd assume that the traumatic experience heart surgery patients go through would be enough incentive to change their habits, especially after being armed with all the dietary information they needed. Not only is this not the case, but there are good reasons why they are unable to make such an important change.

Why *is* it so hard to lose weight and maintain the 'lighter version' of you? Even heart surgery patients seem to struggle. It is almost like there is something in our brain that is holding us back, if not actually driving us to eat more and more.

Indeed, there is. Our brain has been shaped over some four million years by living in a hostile environment. Eating was not a matter of enjoyment but of survival. To understand how your brain works, you have to go back in time....

The benefits of millions of years of practice

While it's unlikely that you spend much time thinking about it, you already know that your brain is much more capable and advanced than a stone-age person's brain. Over hundreds of thousands of years, our brain has developed to help us deal with the more and more complex challenges nature presents us with and with the increasingly complex man-made challenges we create for ourselves.

Think about your ancestors, millions of years ago, and the kind of world they lived in: every day of their life, death was a likely outcome. If they were not killed by a wild animal, there was a fair chance they could die of hunger or be killed by a fellow human. They could freeze to death, drown, die of dehydration in the bright sun or poison themselves by eating the wrong plants. The list of real and present dangers they faced is long.

So what did this wonderful organ, the human brain, do? It developed ingenious ways of keeping our ancestors alive in a hostile environment. The story of human evolution is largely a story of how the brain developed to allow us to deal more effectively with the many threats in our environment, thus increasing our species' chances of survival. The result is an amazing brain that has one major shortcoming: it is not designed for the world most of us live in today....

2

Your 'old' and your 'new' brain

Our brain has developed over thousands of generations and, as it evolved, it became more advanced and could deal with increasingly complex matters.

More specifically, what we might call the 'old brain' developed over a period of some four to five million years. This is a very long time, which has allowed our 'old' brain to become more and more efficient and effective in doing what it does.

So what *does* it do?

The old brain comprises of the emotional part of the brain and controls our hard-wired responses and instincts. It is largely reactive. It is also responsible for habits. Importantly, you are not consciously aware of what your old brain is up to. It works in the non-conscious.

On the other hand, our ability to plan, to look ahead, to analyze and to develop a rational argument are relatively new capabilities, and the areas of the brain responsible for these are located in your frontal lobes, which only developed over the last 80,000 to 100,000 years. This may seem like a long time, but compare that to the 'old' brain, which had some four to five million years to develop.

To put this into perspective, the frontal lobes – the parts that allow you to see yourself in time and space, to plan ahead and to develop a logical argument – have had only around 2 per cent of the time the old brain had to develop. Take a pen and draw a 10-cm-long line. If this is the length of time your old brain had to develop, then 2 mm (*millimeters*, not centimeters!) represents the time your 'new' brain, the frontal lobes, has had time to refine itself.

The result of this imbalance in developmental time is that the older, non-conscious brain is far more advanced and more powerful than the 'new brain'.

You may think of yourself as being smart because you can argue, plan, analyze and make decisions, but it is in fact your older brain – your non-conscious mind – that largely determines what you do.

You may be wondering if I have digressed from our weight loss topic, but I haven't. It is of critical importance for you to understand that your old, emotional brain is much more powerful than your new, rational brain. This is a problem for two reasons: First, your old brain does not understand the decisions you make with your new brain. Second, your old brain is designed to seek immediate rewards.

Problem 1: Having a good reason to change is not enough

When you make a decision to do something, you are using your frontal lobes, i.e., your rational brain. But your old, emotional brain is not influenced by what you decide. In fact, it doesn't even understand what you are on about.

For example, when you think: *I am overweight and at risk of ending up with some serious health problems. I will lose 20 kg to get out of the danger zone*, your old brain understands neither the concept of being overweight nor serious health problems, nor 20kg nor danger zone.

In fact, your rational decision is totally irrelevant to your old brain, which is designed to keep you safe in a hostile environment. Food is essential to survival, so your old brain thinks you are doing well when you are eating. The more you eat, the better, as the old brain is used to a situation where food was scarce and meals certainly not regular. When you eat less or skip a meal, your old brain gets worried: Is there a shortage of food? Is your life under threat?

Your old brain will encourage you to eat to make sure you are surviving and not dying of hunger. It does not understand that in today's environment you are more likely to be at risk from being overweight than from not being able to find food. Your old brain can't think logically and can't analyze and therefore it does not understand how out of place such a response is.

You can decide whatever you want with your new, rational brain, but it will have no impact on your old brain. And, as your old brain is much more powerful and in control of many of the functions that determine how you feel, think and act, it will succeed in driving your behavior regardless of what you decide with your new brain.

Problem 2: Your old brain wants to feel good now

That your old brain doesn't understand the decision you are making with your new brain, i.e., the frontal lobes, is only part of the story. The problem is further complicated by the fact that your old brain is only interested in one thing: immediate rewards!

In fact, we all have a tendency to drift almost automatically towards activities and experiences that are enjoyable while avoiding those that are negative or painful. So, over a period of time, we tend to spend more time and energy on what pleases us and less on what doesn't. This happens without us making an active decision to do so. It is driven by the *natural* desire to repeat good experiences.

This natural tendency to repeat behavior that results in a pleasurable experience served humans well during the earlier stages of our evolution. It was a natural learning process that conditioned us to repeat the behaviors that delivered us benefits. Most life-saving functions, such as breathing, digestion or blood circulation, are regulated by our old brain without us having to think or do anything, but there are a few other things we need to do to survive as individuals or a species, such as eating and procreating. Not surprisingly, to make sure we don't forget these essential investments into our own and our species' future, nature made these activities pleasurable and designed our brain to seek out these experiences.

Unfortunately, in today's world, this drift towards enjoyment and indulgence is often a cause of the very behavior we now want to change. For example, when we enjoy food, we tend to eat a bit more than we should, and when we dislike physical exertion, we tend to give exercise a low priority. This is really quite natural. It is unlikely (though not impossible) for someone who really enjoys physical activity to suffer from a lack of exercise or for someone who doesn't enjoy eating to be overweight.

To summarize the problem, when you decide that you ought to change your behavior, you are essentially working with your new brain. You are being rational. You are deciding to change because you are convinced that there are good reasons for doing so. But *'good for you'* rarely beats *'enjoyable'* as far as your old brain is concerned.

Here are two specific issues that make it difficult to change and then stick with that change:

First, the reward for healthy behavior tends to be delayed. No doubt, losing weight will deliver many health and lifestyle benefits, lift your self-esteem and make you feel more positive about yourself and the world you live in. However, it will take some time for a change in your eating habits to reduce your weight and deliver these benefits.

Unless you enjoy losing weight as such, you won't experience any exciting benefits until later, when your lower weight delivers a happy, healthier you.

For most people, what they have to do to lose weight is not a great experience! In fact, it can make us feel miserable when we can't dig into the food we have come to get used to and expect, or when we have to train ourselves to get used to smaller portion sizes. Our old brain is not likely to accept giving up something enjoyable unless it gets immediate compensation – some immediate feel-good reward. Our old brain doesn't listen to reason; it simply wants to feel good.

Second, the benefits are sometimes intangible. '*Good for you*' sometimes means that we want to make a change to avoid something bad happening later in life. In other words, the reward is that something bad that could happen is less likely to happen.

For example, a key reason for wanting to lose weight may be that you want to avoid health problems later on, but giving up the pleasure of eating food you like (and lots of it too!) doesn't provide your old brain with a tangible, immediate benefit. You are likely to find that your old brain is reluctant to trade today's enjoyment to avoid something (as bad as it might be) that *may or may not* happen at some time in the future.

It isn't that your old brain is rejecting the deal you are offering it, but rather that it doesn't even understand the deal. Your old brain is instinctive and on the lookout for rewards, and when you feel like a great hamburger, chocolate bar or pile of waffles, your old brain really wants to have it – right there and then.

All this adds up to a more than unsatisfactory situation. We may succeed in changing our eating behaviors at first, because we feel good about being able to make a positive change. We feel in charge, competent, maybe even righteous, because we are succeeding at making a change we believe is important.

The initial success allows us to feel successful and good about ourselves. But, as soon as this initial self-congratulatory phase is over, our old brain seeks out the enjoyment our old behaviors used to deliver, and it seeks to eliminate the frustration our new regime is causing. When we reach that point, our old brain will try to take us back to our old ways of behaving.

In summary, a rational decision to change our behavior and the resulting intention is quite ineffective in getting our old brain on board. Unfortunately, however, to be successful, we *do* need both brains to get on board.

I expect that these insights into how our brain works line up with your own personal experience: whenever you have made changes that resulted in immediate pleasure, with no down-side, you most likely found it easy to maintain the new behaviors. You may have found it quite easy to make time for a television series you wanted to watch regularly, or to get off the couch to pick up the take-away dinner you enjoy so much.

But when sacrifices need to be made without the compensation of immediate rewards, the change we decide to put in place is difficult to make and to sustain. While it doesn't seem so hard to make time for a television series you want to watch, you find all sorts of excuses when it comes to changing your eating habits or making time for exercise.

The most difficult changes are those that are sensible from a rational point of view but that require you to change your behavior without offering strong, immediate emotional rewards for doing so. These are the changes we typically struggle with – and losing weight is one of them!

Conclusion

Today, we may think of ourselves as rational beings that can not only make decisions but also carry them out simply by sticking with them. However, we are often surprised to find that this is not the way our brains really work.

Yes, the human brain is a highly sophisticated organ – in fact, it's the most advanced organ we know of, and far more powerful than the most powerful computer we can build. It not only regulates the processes that keep you alive, it also develops absolutely ingenious ways of protecting you.

Therein, however, lies the major problem: your brain was designed to protect and serve you *in the hostile environments of our past*. Many of the responses your brain has developed and refined over millions of years are not particularly useful in today's environment.

Given that you are reading this book, I can safely assume that you don't live in a hostile natural environment where your brain must focus on keeping you safe. You don't have to hunt for food, and you can have your next meal whenever you want to. However, your old brain doesn't know that. It assumes that you still live in a hostile environment, and so it continues to act in the way it knows best – it's goal is to protect you, to keep you safe, and to increase your chances of survival.

By doing so, it actually puts you at risk in the environment you live in today. It makes it difficult for you to give up bad eating habits. It makes it difficult for you to make changes that would improve your health and your quality of life.

There is nothing wrong with you if you find it difficult to lose weight. Your old brain is not designed to help you with conscious dietary changes or other conscious changes. Rather, it will obstruct change through the very processes that helped humankind to survive in the hostile environment of long ago.

However, the situation is not hopeless. Armed with this understanding we can develop a weight loss program that is aligned with the way our brain works rather than simply ignore this formidable barrier and assume that all we need to do is go on a diet and stick with it. I will present a number of effective strategies to reach and maintain a Happy Weight. Before we get to that, there are a few more important barriers to success you need to know about.

3
We are creatures of habit

In the previous chapter, I covered three limitations of your old brain:

1   It can't understand a rational argument.

2   It's only objective is to keep you alive and safe.

3   It wants immediate rewards.

Now I want to add a fourth limitation:

4   You are a creature of habit.

As we've already seen, most of our brain evolved over some four or five million years, and this old brain has mastered a hugely useful trick: it can turn repeat behavior into a routine that can be played out without any conscious thought.

Let me start with an example: Remember when you were learning to drive a car (or, if you don't drive, remember some other highly challenging task like learning to play golf or ride a bicycle). While you were learning, you were most likely focusing consciously on what you needed to do: when to apply the brakes and how hard, when and how to change gears, when and how to use the indicator in time for your next turn, when to look behind you before changing lanes, and so on.

For most of us, learning how to drive was quite stressful and we had to give it our full attention to be able to cope with the multitude of tasks and new challenges we faced. After all, the road is a complex environment with lots of often unpredictable things happening at once.

However, once you got more and more used to driving, you most likely started to give this activity less and less of your full attention. Driving eventually became routinized or 'automated'.

You no longer had to consciously plan each move you made, because you could let your non-conscious mind – your old brain – take over.

This means that most of the actions you now take when driving are triggered by your mind without you even being aware of it. Driving probably feels more and more like something you do 'automatically', with no need to focus your attention on *how* to drive except when something new and unexpected comes up.

The same applies to just about anything we do regularly that does not require deviations from the normal patterns – from brushing our teeth to having a shower, starting the computer to picking groceries off the shelves in the supermarket. We are on automatic pilot, so to speak.

Letting your non-conscious mind take care of repetitive activities is, of course, a very important part of the way our brain works. If we couldn't let our non-conscious mind take over the activities we have already learnt, we wouldn't be able to do more than one thing at a time, because our conscious attention can't focus on more than one thing at once.

To go back to our driving example, because your brain has allowed your non-conscious mind to take over the routine task of driving, you can now drive *and* have a chat with a passenger, think about what to have for dinner, or plan what you need to do at work today. How clever is that? I am always amazed by how the human brain has developed to allow us to do many things simultaneously with greater ease!

Are you increasing the risk of an accident by letting your non-conscious take over? I would argue that you are in fact *reducing* the risk of an accident. Your conscious mind is quite slow and not capable of dealing with complex situations.

Your non-conscious mind, on the other hand, is able to deal with complex situations at lightning speed, as long as there are relevant past experiences stored as memories it can draw on. It follows the routines you have learned so it can free up your conscious mind for more interesting, important or enjoyable pursuits.

In summary, habits are learned behaviors, and learning is simply creating memories of 'how to do it' through repetitive behavior. Once you've had enough experience of a behavior, you can leave it to your non-conscious mind to take over. The non-conscious mind relies on the massive bank of memories that has been built by repeating this behavior again and again.

Now, imagine for a minute what life would be like if we didn't have a non-conscious mind to take over the activities we have learnt to the extent that they have become routinized. We would have to give our full attention to everything we do. This would obviously limit our capacity to get things done.

If we had to give every activity our full attention, it is doubtful that anyone would ever have invented the motor car or supermarkets. Our ability to routinize what we do frees up our minds for other challenges, and this has been a key factor in the evolution of the human species and in the way we now live our lives.

However, there is also a severe downside to our natural tendency to form automatic habits: once we have learned to do certain things habitually and do them in a particular way, we find it very hard to change these behaviors. Even when we make a conscious decision to change by using our rational new brain, our non-conscious mind located in our old brain will take us back to our established habits.

In summary, habitual behaviors are great because they allow us to give our attention to other more rewarding matters while our non-conscious mind runs the bits of our life that are really just repeats. But this same habitualization becomes a problem when we want to change the habits that have formed over time, such as our eating habits.

4
Why diets don't work

Neuroscience has allowed us to learn increasingly more about how our brain works, and one of the insights we have gained is an understanding of why diets don't work. In this chapter, I will explore this issue in greater depth.

When referring to a 'diet' in everyday language – as in, 'I am going on a diet' – we are typically referring to an unbalanced eating regime designed to help us shed some weight. Unbalanced diets of this nature do not reflect what a healthy person should eat long-term. They intentionally deviate from what is a healthy food intake for the average person to allow the dieter to meet a short-term weight goal.

It should therefore come as no surprise to learn that these diets don't work.

Of course, anyone can shed a few kilos when eliminating carbohydrates, or when eating only grapefruit, or protein, or broccoli, or grapes, or whatever the latest diet fad suggests. But these diets are not only unhealthy, they can't deliver weight maintenance.

For example, when you go on an Atkins diet, you are going

to lose weight – no doubt about it. But if you stay on this diet for too long, you are likely to damage your organs, especially your liver. The Atkins diet, like many other diets, is designed to induce (usually rapid) weight loss, not to get you used to a long-term eating regime that will allow you to keep the excess weight off.

The problem is that when you get off the diet, you still haven't developed great eating habits that will serve you for the rest of your life. This is why the vast majority of people can't maintain the weight loss they achieved while on a diet.

It is better not to diet at all than to put the weight back on later

Given that diets provide short-term weight loss only, it may look like a neat solution to go on a diet, lose weight, and then go back on the diet later, after the weight has returned. In other words, it may seem that you must accept that you will be going through a cycle of dieting – diet, weight loss, weight gain, diet, weight loss, weight gain, diet, and so forth – for the rest of your life.

This would allow you to keep your weight reasonably close to your goal weight. But it would also bankrupt your health.

Losing weight and putting it back on is worse than not losing it at all, because when you lose weight you shed muscle tissue as well as fat cells. When you put the weight back on, your body only generates fat cells, so you end up less healthy than you were before you embarked on this weight-loss adventure.

If going on a diet and maintaining a lower weight afterwards typically doesn't work, and if the *'diet, lose weight, stop diet, gain weight, diet again'* merry-go-round is worse for you than not losing weight in the first place, what's left?

Focus not on eating but on what drives you to eat!

Here is an obvious solution: adopt a healthy-eating regime you can get used to and maintain for the rest of your life! *'Great,'* I hear you mutter, *'I have bought a book that tells me the obvious. I've tried this before and couldn't make it stick'*

The problem is that you are likely to have some Eating Drivers that keep pushing you to eat more. Let me use a simple example to explain what I mean before turning my attention to your weight loss challenge.

Imagine a father who seems unable to find enough time to spend with his children. One day, he decides to rectify the situation: *'I will spend more time with my children,'* he says to himself. *'I don't want to miss being part of their lives when they grow up!'* The following diagram shows the assessment this father made (the two boxes) and the decision he reached (the bubble below). This all makes good sense.

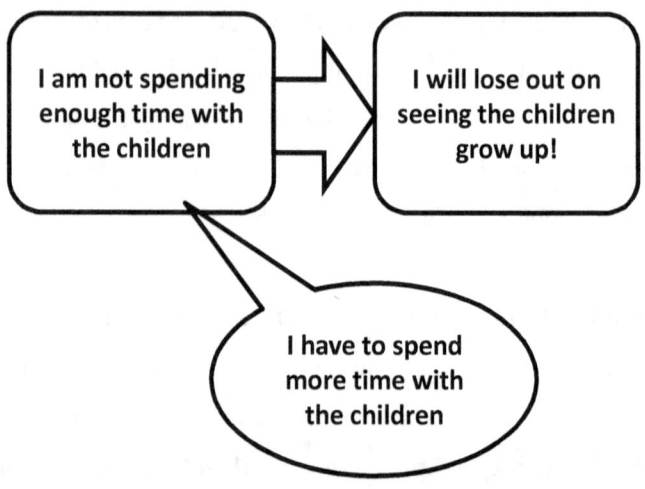

This is surely a reasonable approach to changing the way he lives his life. He has looked at how little time he spends with his children and has made a sound decision to spend more time with them. However, after initially sticking to his decision, he quickly falls back into his earlier pattern of simply running out of time and being unable to give much of what precious time is left over to his children.

The point is that he is unlikely to succeed unless he identifies and addresses the Drivers that cause him to spend time elsewhere. The key question he needs to ask himself is this: '*Why* am I spending too little time with my children?'

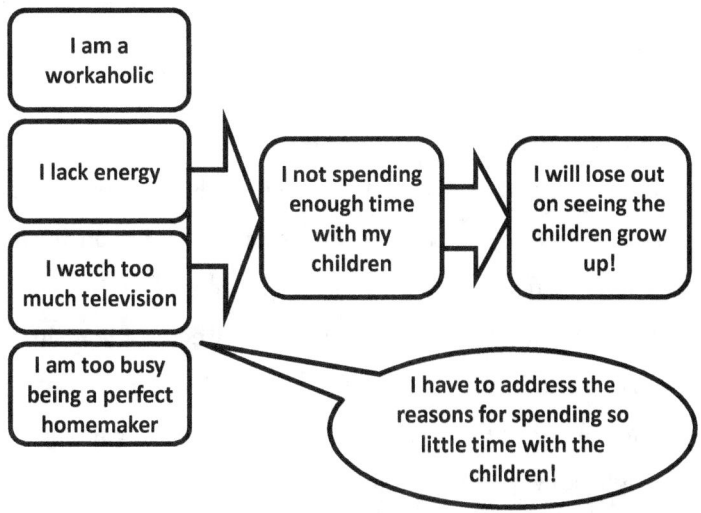

Is it because I spend too much time working? Or because I lack energy to give them my attention by the time I am free? Or do I tend to drift off into other activities such as watching television? Or am I a perfectionist who simply can't let matters go and focus on what's really important to me – being with my children – because I first have to finish off everything perfectly, all the time?

There could be all sorts of reasons. Making a decision to change behavior without addressing your personal Drivers is not likely to succeed. I am sure you will agree and join me in suggesting to this father that making the decision to spend more time with his children is not going to be enough to make it happen. Rather, he will have to work out the *reasons* for giving so little time to his children and then work on dealing with these barriers to success.

Let's get back to your weight challenge. To be successful, you too will need to identify, understand and deal with your reasons for overeating and for eating the wrong foods. It is not enough to assume that all you need to do is make a decision to lose weight and then somehow you will be able to stick with it.

Naturally, you *would* succeed in losing weight if you simply ate less and ate different foods. But if a simple decision was enough – if it were that easy – you would not be reading this book right now, and we would not find that more than half of the people in developed countries are overweight!

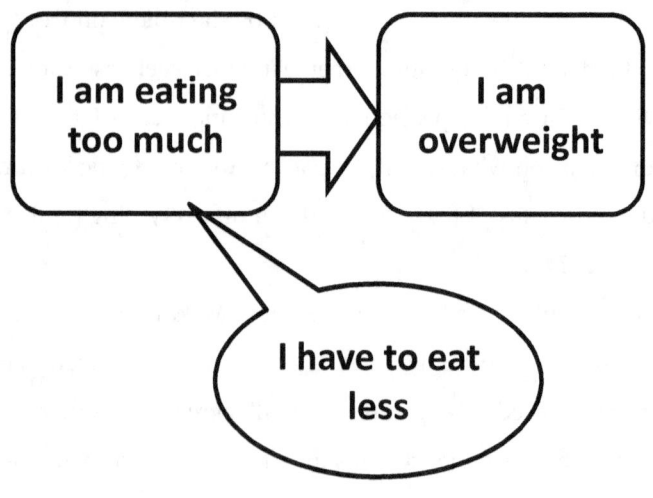

You have reasons for eating too much, and unless you address these reasons you are not likely to succeed. First there are Eating Drivers. There are all the factors that push you to eat more and to eat unhealthy foods and that, by doing so, make it extremely difficult for you to change your eating behavior.

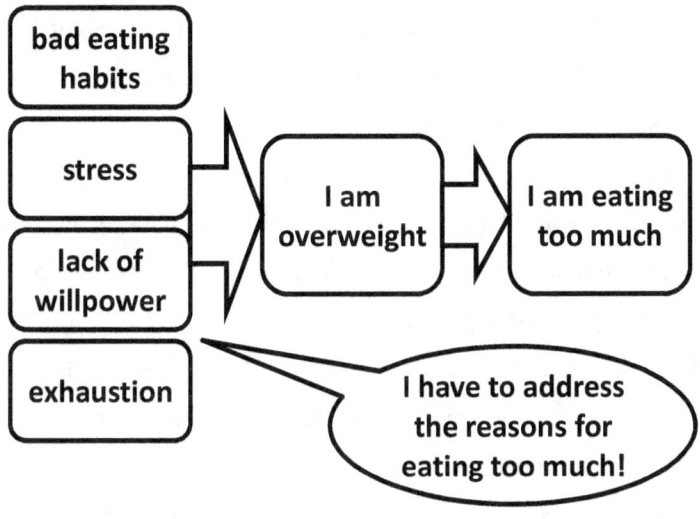

Second, there are the barriers to making a change. We have covered quite a few already: the fact that your non-conscious mind, which controls your desire to eat, does not understand a rational argument for losing weight; your non-conscious mind, wanting immediate rewards, is unprepared to wait for the many benefits a reduced weight might deliver in a few months; and the difficulty in changing bad eating habits once they have become well-established in your non-conscious mind.

I have one strong message I'd like to make clear here: If you *don't* deal with these Eating Drivers and the Barriers to Change, you are *unlikely* to succeed. This has been evidenced by tens if not hundreds of millions of people who thought all they needed to do is to go on a diet. You may lose some weight initially on a diet, but it is unlikely that you can maintain your weight loss. You must deal with your Eating Drivers and Barriers to Change to lose weight and maintain this weight loss.

In addition to this, you also need to learn what and how much you should be eating, especially if you don't already know much about food and nutrition. Many of us have no idea as to what an appropriate portion size is or what foods we should eat. More often than not, this is not due to a lack of information but rather the consequence of having too much (and often conflicting) information.

In other words, you not only need to deal with the root causes that lead you to overeat and/or eat the wrong foods, you must also learn the skills necessary to make healthy food-choices and to understand how much should be eaten at what time. The latter is, in my experience, the easier part; but regardless of how easy or hard it is, you are well advised to start by weakening or even eliminating your Eating Drivers.

5

The Seven Golden Rules

Golden Rule No 1:
Don't do anything you can't maintain long term!

This is the most important rule. There is no point in pushing ahead and making progress quickly when you can't maintain your Happy Weight in the end. As you already know, losing weight and putting it back on is worse for your health than not losing it in the first place. Add to this the frustration you will surely experience when you find that you can't maintain your weight and end up back where you started, or in an even worse position.

The right approach is to think about your weight loss as a journey that takes place over a long period of time. You need to make progress in small stages – small enough for you to be able to maintain any weight loss you have achieved.

I am stating the obvious here, but dieters don't seem to consider this fact: if you lose (say) ten kilograms in six weeks and put that weight back on within a year, you are much worse off than if you had lost just a couple of kilos and then grown used to the change in lifestyle that allowed you to do this.

Maybe four weeks later you would have been ready to lose another two kilos and settle down again at your new lower weight before losing more.

If it took you a couple of weeks to lose two kilos and then four weeks to get used to maintaining your new weight, it would take you a total of 26 weeks to reach your Happy Weight (i.e., a loss of ten kilograms in total, after spending ten weeks losing weight and 16 weeks to periodically focus on maintaining your weight loss after each 2-kg step).

Yes, you could have gotten to the same lower weight in six weeks if you had not paid attention to maintaining your lower weight in stages, but in scenario 1 you would most likely put the weight back on within a year. In scenario 2, it might take you nearly eight months to reach your Happy Weight, but you will be able to maintain this weight for the rest of your life. Which is the better outcome?

Here are some guidelines for how to approach your weight loss:

- Don't develop a long-term program that specifies now how much weight you should lose over the next few weeks or months. Your challenge is to learn how to *maintain* any weight loss. Once you have learned to manage that, you can slowly lose weight and, by simply maintaining your position until you are used to it, you can move onto the next stage and eventually, can reach any goal you want. There is no point locking yourself into a long-term program with fixed timeframes when you don't know how long it will take you to learn weight maintenance.

- Don't set ambitious targets. Again, the focus is on maintenance. It is much better to lose just a couple of kilos and then switch to maintaining this lower weight than to aim at a more significant weight loss which you are unlikely to be able to maintain. Set a moderate goal to start with, and then use some of the techniques I cover later in the book to learn to maintain your weight loss.

As the title of this book suggests, you need to find your Happy Weight, i.e., the weight that is right for you. Your Happy Weight allows you to have the energy and flexibility to do the things you want to do and eliminates any worries about weight-related health issues down the track.

It's unlikely you know what your Happy Weight is, unless you have been at this weight for an extended period and feel really well, energetic and able to live life to the fullest.

You can look up a BMI (Body Mass Index) table on the internet and find what your 'ideal weight' is, but keep in mind that this ideal weight is only an approximation anyway. I feel it is much more important for you to discover your Happy Weight by learning to lose weight successfully, but slowly. When you reach your Happy Weight, you will know it – you will feel great and you will want to maintain that weight.

It follows that you should not set yourself an end point when you are just starting out. Instead, simply focus on losing a bit of weight, and then switch to maintenance until you are sure you can preserve the weight loss you have made. Only at that point should you switch back to losing weight. If you embrace this cycle, you will one day find that you are really happy with your weight and are able to manage it easily. That's when you have found your Happy Weight! As you grow older or get used to carrying less weight, you may well revise your Happy Weight, but that should be no problem as by then you will be very good at weight maintenance and will find it easy to adjust your weight without having to work too hard on it.

Golden Rule No 2:
Learn to make your 'old' brain feel good!

As discussed earlier, your old brain does not understand reason. It therefore can't buy into your plan to reach and maintain your Happy Weight. Your old brain wants you to eat a lot to make sure you don't die of hunger, because it is designed to keep you alive in a hostile environment. And it wants immediate rewards.

Your challenge is to allow your old brain to experience the benefits of reaching and maintaining your Happy Weight by imagining them.

When this technique is used in sports psychology, the focus

is on visualizing the emotional rewards of winning. In our case, it is a matter of visualizing the emotional rewards of succeeding, i.e., how great you will feel when you have reached your Happy Weight and are able to maintain it without feeling deprived or needing to make an effort.

It is important that you don't just imagine the actual outcome, but the positive emotions you will feel when you achieve this outcome. These are the rewards your old brain is seeking, and the rewards it will eventually experience as a result of the changes you are planning to make.

You should embellish these rewards in your mind as much as possible. Go into great detail visualizing how great you will feel to be finally free of this burden, how great you will feel when you've taken charge of your own destiny, how great you will feel telling a friend about your successful change, and so on.

If you feel uncomfortable doing something like this, remember that your imagination can trigger the same processes in your brain that take place when you experience the real thing. For example, experiments have shown that people who visualize doing physical exercise *do* build some muscle strength, although not as much as people who actually undertake these exercises, of course.

You probably know from your own experience that imagining something really sad makes you feel sad, while imagining something positive and happy lifts your spirits. In these and other cases, the brain is tricked into releasing the same hormones and neurotransmitters it would release in a real-world situation. Once those chemicals are released, the impact on your body and mind is much the same, whether the situation is real or imaginary.

I recommend that you take the visualization exercise seriously. Sit down, close your eyes, and go through a relaxation exercise to get you into the right space, and then imagine the emotional benefits in as much detail as you can. See yourself, hear yourself, see and hear the reactions of others. It is important for you to do this regularly, especially whenever you experience a relapse into your old habits. The added benefit is that a relaxed visualization session in itself is a great way to feel calmer and better!

Here is an illustration of what a visualization session might look like. Clearly you have to focus on the emotional benefits of weight loss that are important to you, so I am not suggesting you follow the 'script' below. But this illustration may be useful if you are not familiar with visualization.

Ideally, start with a relaxation session (you will find guidelines for conducting a relaxation session in Chapter 11: Living without stress). Once you are relaxed, start to visualize your success - when you have reached a milestone on your weight journey...

• imagine how you will feel

- feel your self-confidence

- feel the energy you have

- feel the excitement that comes from reaching this milestone

- now imagine what you can do (once you reach this milestone) that you find difficult to do right now

- imagine how you will be active - what exactly are you going to do

- imagine the response of others that are close to you - family, friends, colleagues

- imagine details - like what people would be saying

- imagine the occasions - where are you, what else is happening there, what are people doing,...

- feel how great it is to be supported and acknowledged by these people who are close to you

- imaging doing things you wanted to do for a long time, but did not or were not able to do -

  - may be going to the beach with confidence

  - may be going out

  - may be making love

  - may be trying on some clothes that didn't fit you any more

  - may be buying some new clothes

- just imagine as many good things you will be able to do as you can think off - spend time with each one, bring the occasion alive, feel the excitement and satisfaction, feel the reward for all your hard work...

- When you have finished take your time and enjoy feeling great before you open your eyes.

Don't use fear to motivate yourself

It is important that you focus on the *positive*, not the negative. Remember the heart patients? They didn't change their behavior, despite the significant threat to their health and even to their lives.

Fear is not a great motivator. Every day that passes without the feared consequences eventuating confirms in your mind that you are okay, despite the potential long-term problems you may face one day. In other words, every day that goes by without any negative consequences will strengthen your old brain's focus on immediate benefits by convincing you that 'the bad stuff won't happen to me anyway'.

If you use fear regularly in your visualization, you can expect to create a rather depressed and negative mindset.

In summary, don't focus on losing weight to avoid health problems that might occur when you are older (which is about fear). Instead, focus on the benefits you will gain: feeling more attractive, breathing more easily, being able to do whatever it is you want to do, having more energy, experiencing a lift in self-confidence, et cetera.

Rule No3:
Be good to your body while you fix your mind!

There are a number of things you should attempt to do as much of as you can. Don't get frustrated if you find it difficult or if you don't fall into a regular habit for a while.

Here are some specific suggestions:

Get enough sleep

Unfortunately, many people don't get enough sleep these days. A study conducted by the National Sleep Foundation in 2008 showed that American adults get some two hours of sleep less per night than they did in 1960.

Studies show that there are several promising strategies you can employ: a single good night's sleep will restore your brain function; getting enough sleep early in the week might allow you to build up a reserve that counteracts sleep deprivation later in the week; taking a short nap can make a world of difference when you are overtired. Other research suggests that it's the number of consecutive hours you spend awake that matters most - so try to avoid unnaturally long periods without any sleep. Kelly McGonical suggests you try one of these strategies: catching up, stocking up or napping.[1]

---

[1] McGonical Kelly, *The Willpower Instinct: How Self-Control Works, Why It Matters and What You Can Do to Get More of It,* New York 2012, p. 47

Eat more...

Finally, I want you to eat something healthy, in a reasonable quantity, every day. You probably think I am mad asking you to eat more when you are trying to lose weight, but don't worry; there is a specific reason for this request: your brain will encourage you to eat until the most important minerals, vitamins, proteins and carbohydrates have been ingested. By eating some healthy food, you may find your appetite is reduced. Research has shown that many people reduce the amount of unhealthy food they used to eat regularly once they start including something healthy in their diet. This reduction is without their conscious effort; it simply happens automatically.

Ideally, add some foods with a low glycemic index. This includes *nuts, most vegetables, many raw fruits, cheese, fish, meat, olive oil and other 'good' fats.* These foods will also help you to gain more energy, feel less tired and maintain your glucose level better.

When you consume alcohol, do it in moderation

Alcohol is best consumed in moderation not only because most alcoholic drinks put a lot of calories into your body but also because alcohol causes a lack of self-control. When you drink, you start to lose your ability to monitor your own behavior. In this state, it is natural to simply eat whatever you feel like – and lots of it!

I am not suggesting you should give up alcohol if you enjoy the occasional drink - just be aware of its potential to upset your weight loss journey and try to drink in moderation or only on special occasions.

Rule No4:
Decide up-front which bad habits you are not going to change!

It is quite common for people who try to lose weight to set themselves specific eating targets. Some dieters count calories, some have pre-portioned meal sizes, and others follow a menu list or have a specific eating plan in mind.

When dieters exceed their planned food intake quite dramatically for some unexpected reason (for example, because they feel particularly stressed and indulge in comfort food, or they are exhausted and use food to get more energy, or because they have a long lunch with friends and end up eating much more than planned...), they regard their diet as blown for the day and continue to eat excessively – and this resulting binge often causes them to put on far more weight than the original lapse would have. Also, once they have broken their diet, they become less aware of what they are eating....[2]

You should preempt such a reaction by deciding now, up-

---

[2] Baumeister, Roy F. and John Tierney, *Willpower: Rediscovering the Greatest Human Strength,* The Penguin Press, New York, 2011, pp 221–222

front, on what occasions you will allow yourself to indulge. For argument's sake, let's say you have a meal with friends once or twice a month and you really enjoy their company and eating and drinking is a big part of this occasion. You can decide right now that you will not change this part of your life. I am sure there are plenty of other aspects of your life you can change to reach your Happy Weight, so there is nothing wrong with making a decision to keep some of the less healthy habits going.

However, there are two provisos you should first consider:

First, refuse to maintain a bad habit that is frequent in nature. You might decide to eat and drink as much as you want once or twice a month when you meet up with your friends, but do not decide to keep eating unhealthy foods in large quantities while watching television every day. Clearly, anything you do frequently that has a negative impact on your weight needs to be changed; whereas, any times of indulgence that you really treasure and that are infrequent you can allow yourself to continue with.

Second, you need to make an upfront decision about what you are changing and what infrequent situations will be exempt from change. Do not allow yourself to include additional eating occasions at a later stage.

You have to decide now what is excluded from your effort to reach a Happy Weight. Write it down so there is no uncertainty later on. And make sure you only exclude something that is really important to you and does not occur frequently.

Rule No 5:
Know where you are on your journey

There is an old saying 'What you measure is what you get!' Measuring something makes it visible and focuses your mind on whatever it **is**. When you weigh yourself every day, you are constantly reminding yourself of your plan to lose weight and at the same time getting immediate feedback that tells you where on your journey you are.

If you like, you can use self-quantification software, which is available free of charge on various websites such as Stickk.com.

But whatever you do, make sure you ask yourself the right question! When people who have taken a positive step toward meeting a goal think in terms of how much progress they make, they are more likely to do something that conflicts with their goal; for example, they may skip the gym next day or overindulge when eating.

In contrast, people who think in terms of how committed they feel to their goal are rarely tempted by conflicting behaviors.

Let me illustrate this by referring to a study carried out by the Hong Kong University of Science and the University of Chicago: students were asked to remember a time they turned down a temptation. After doing this, 70 percent of the participants took the next opportunity to indulge. This is due to 'moral licensing,' which is the process that leads your mind to demand a reward for having succeeded at a difficult task. In other words, when you see that you have lost some weight, moral licensing would encourage you to eat because you deserve a reward for having been so good.

When the researchers asked participants in this study to remember *why* they had resisted, the licensing disappeared – 69 per cent resisted temptation. Remembering the *why* works because it puts your focus on your goal and also reinforces the goal, rather than suggesting that you have done well and thus deserve a reward.[3]

In addition to measuring your weight, you should also make it a habit to measure your portion sizes. It is good practice to pay attention to portion sizes and, if appropriate, start using a smaller plate as a means of making you aware of how much you should eat. Research has shown that when food is served on large plates and when drinks are served in large glasses, we tend to underestimate how much we consume.

Rule No 6:
Don't be tricked by low-fat, organic or healthy menu items !

---

[3] McGonical Kelly, *The Willpower Instinct: How Self-Control Works, Why It Matters and What You Can Do to Get More of It*, New York 2012, p.90–91

Studies show that people who eat a healthy meal - or even just a healthy dish as part of a meal - are more likely to go on to consume indulgent drinks, side dishes, desserts, or snacks. In the end they consume more calories than people who did not have a healthy meal or dish at all. They overestimate the contribution their healthy choice has made and, given the healthy food they had, feel that they can now afford to add some less healthy options.

Researchers have also found that people typically estimate that a cheeseburger with a green salad has fewer calories than the same cheeseburger served by itself.[4] It is interesting that even nutritional experts seem to fall for this quite often: they too often underestimate the calories in low-fat or organic foods.

Don't drink diet drinks

I need to warn you of the impact of diet drinks such as Diet Coke, Coke Zero or Pepsi Max. The sweet taste of these drinks suggests to the brain that there will be a sugar spike, and, in response, the body takes up loads of glucose from the bloodstream to compensate for the coming spike. However, the spike never arrives, because these drinks use artificial sweeteners rather than sugar. As a result, you end up with low glucose and less energy. As crazy as it may seem, these diet sodas contribute to overeating and weight gain.

---

[4] McGonical Kelly, ibid., p.99–100

Rule No7:
Don't try too many things at the same time!

There is no point in trying a dozen actions that address various weight-related problems if it will only make you tired, confused, and frustrated. Trying to change too much at once can be very ineffective. Start with a change you feel confident you can make and sustain. Once you have made that change move on to some of the most critical actions you need to take – i.e., those that will have the greatest long-term impact and provide a sound foundation for you to build on as you move on – and don't try to do everything at once. If you do, my prediction is that ultimately you will fail.

Summary – the Seven Golden Rules

1. Don't do anything you can't maintain long term.
2. Learn to make your old brain feel good.
3. Be good to your body while you fix your mind.
4. Decide up-front which bad habits you are not going to change.
5. Know where you are on your journey.
6. Don't be tricked by low-fat, organic or healthy menu items.
7. Don't try too many things at the same time.

You may already follow some of these rules. Maybe you already eat largely healthy food and get enough sleep, or you already spend time visualizing the benefits of reaching your Happy Weight. However, in other instances you might have to take some action. As I said before, don't turn this into a high-stress exercise. Give yourself time to introduce the changes necessary for you to be able to follow these Golden Rules.

The one technique that may take some time to learn is visualization; however, I very strongly suggest you give it the time it deserves. This is an important technique to learn and refine, as it is the most effective way to influence your old brain. Once you master visualization, you will have some very rewarding visualization sessions, with the great benefit that your mind will allow you to lose weight and to maintain your Happy Weight.

Follow these Golden Rules until your new behaviors are automatic, i.e., they become habits. In doing so, you will have built a solid foundation to now address the other major challenges you face, from changing your bad eating habits to eliminating stress from your life.

The next step...

The second part of this book is designed to help you to turn bad eating habits into good ones, to boost your willpower, and to eliminate chronic stress from your life. However, my advice is not to rush on from here. It is important that you give yourself time to explore the Seven Golden Rules and to take action where required.

If there is more than one area where you need to make a change, you should take a step-by-step approach, starting with an easy change and only moving onto the next challenge once you are confident you can maintain your recently changed behavior.

Addressing habits, dealing with stress and boosting your willpower are all important, but you will be in a much stronger position to address these major challenges once you live by the Seven Golden Rules and laid a solid foundation for change.

PART II
The big issues

6

More about habits

In this section we will focus on how to turn bad eating habits into good ones.

More specifically,

- *how habits are formed,*
- *what triggers our habits into action,*
- *how we can disrupt our habits.*

Armed with a clear understanding of our habits, we can develop a personalized program for turning our bad eating habits into good ones.

How habits are formed

Rather than tell you how your brain is sabotaging your best efforts to lose and then maintain your weight, I want you to play a game. The rules are very simple: I will tell you a story that describes a person in a prehistoric situation and then ask you what sort of a response you would want to build into that person's brain to help her in that situation. I know it sounds silly, but I promise it will be instructive!

Stories from another time: Herkja's Story

Herkja is carting the berries and roots the tribe has collected and the handicrafts they have laboriously created to the next village, to trade them for tools and meat. As always, when balancing her heavy load on the top of her head, she has to give her full attention to the task, just like when she weaves cloth or searches for roots. A lack of concentration could limit what she has to trade with or, worse, lead to a loss of the little she has found.

Here is your question: *What would you ideally want Herkja's brain to do to help her make progress?*

Here is what her brain *will* do for her: it will allow her to develop habits, i.e., to automatically repeat behaviors that she performs often.

If she continues to engage in a repetitive behavior, her brain will eventually learn to repeat this behavior without her having to give it any conscious attention. This will free up her 'thinking' brain to work out better ways of harvesting berries and roots, create new handicrafts, or to bring these to the market.

While it is not likely that she will come up with a breakthrough invention like the wheel, she might well adapt some of the basic tools she uses to make them more effective or to reduce the effort required when using them. Without her brain's ability to habitualize, she would not be able to give her attention to developing such improvements; all her attention would be focused on carrying out repetitive tasks.

The brain has found an absolutely amazing way to contribute to human progress in this hostile and difficult environment. But is habitualizing a double-edged sword in today's world? In Herkja's time, humans had to focus on what was important to their survival, and habitualizing repetitive tasks allowed them to address more of the other challenges they faced. Today, habitualization is still very useful because it allows us to get much more done, but we are just as likely to habitualize bad behaviors, such as poor eating habits, as we are good behaviors. This is a problem because habits are very difficult to break once they have been established.

How we develop habits

Let me go back to our driving example. While you were learning, you were focusing consciously on what you needed to do: when to apply the brakes and how hard, when and how to change gears, when and how to use the indicator in time for your next turn, when to look behind you before changing lanes, and so on.

However, once you got more and more used to driving, you most likely started to give this activity less and less of your full attention. Driving eventually became routinized or 'automated'.

You no longer had to consciously plan each move you made,

because you could let your non-conscious mind take over.

Similarly, when we learn a sport, language or instrument, we learn by repetition – by building memory patterns that then allow us to act without thinking. Martial arts training is a great example of this principle: the repetition of movements imprints these actions on the mind, ready to be called on automatically whenever a situation demands it. If you had to pause to think about what to do when attacked, you would react too late to successfully ward off the attack. Repeating these behaviors to imprint them eliminates the need to consciously think about what to do, which is especially important when fast reactions are required.

To go back to our driving example, because your brain has allowed your non-conscious mind to take over the routine task of driving, you can now drive *and* have a chat with a passenger, think about what to have for dinner, or plan what you need to do at work today. How clever is that? I am always amazed by how the human brain has developed to allow us to do more things simultaneously with greater ease!

Getting your non-conscious mind to take over: Repeat triggers

There are many activities you probably do automatically, from making a cup of tea or coffee or washing the dishes to walking to work or turning on the computer in the morning. But how does your non-conscious mind know when to take over? How does it know to engage in driving behavior only when you are in your car but not when you are in bed? Why don't you wake up at night only to find yourself sitting up in bed and acting out driving motions?

The answer is that there are so-called repeat triggers that activate particular habits. Your non-conscious mind learned to associate these triggers with certain behaviors, because in the past the behaviors always followed these certain triggers.

For example, you walk up to your car and take out your keys before you get in and drive. So, as you learn how to drive, your non-conscious mind begins connecting your approach to the car and the preparations for driving (including unlocking the door, putting the key into the ignition, putting on the seatbelt, and whatever else you do every time to get ready to drive) with the driving behaviors that always follow.

Similarly, when certain items or activities always (or at least often) precede eating, your non-conscious mind connects these cues with the following eating behaviors. If you regularly eat snacks when sitting on the couch to watch television, your non-conscious mind learns that couch+television is followed by food, which means that when you sit down and turn the television on, you will feel driven to eat something.

Alerting your conscious mind: Alert triggers

Your conscious mind is quite slow and not capable of dealing with complex situations. In the example of driving, I have argued that rather than increasing the risk of an accident by letting your non-conscious take over when you drive, you are in fact *reducing* the risk of an accident, because your non-conscious mind is able to deal with complex situations at lightning speed, as long as there are relevant past experiences stored as memories it can draw on. It takes care of routine behaviors in order to free up your conscious mind for more interesting, important or enjoyable pursuits.

What your non-conscious mind is not good at, however, is dealing with *new situations* where there are *no* past experiences in your memory to draw on. This is understandable because your non-conscious relies on your past experience to decide what needs to be done.

When you learn to drive, your non-conscious mind busily creates memories of road situations and the appropriate driving behavior, and once you have a vast collection of driving memories and have habitualized driving, your non-conscious mind can take over and constantly monitor what is happening on the road. As long as the situation is consistent with your memory patterns, it can manage driving very well. You can even have an interesting chat with a passenger or listen intently to the news while driving.

However, when an unusual situation like an accident scene appears ahead of you, your non-conscious mind may not be able to find any relevant memories that help to determine how you should deal with this situation. At this point in time, your non-conscious mind alerts your conscious mind to this unusual situation, and your conscious mind takes over.

This allows you to consciously think about how you might deal with this unusual situation. It also means that you have to stop whatever else you have been were doing besides driving, because your conscious mind can't give full attention to more than one activity at a time.

The important point here is that you don't have to *consciously* decide to change focus: your non-conscious mind simply calls on your conscious mind as soon as an out-of-the-ordinary situation comes up.

The same thing happens when you go to pick up your usual brand of coffee at the supermarket and discover it's out of stock, or when you rent an unfamiliar car that requires you to think about how to start it and where the various levers and buttons are. Your conscious mind must take over for you to successfully navigate these new situations.

Why habits are so strong

Imagine for a minute what life would be like if we didn't have a non-conscious mind to take over the activities we have learnt to the extent that they have become routinized; we would have to give our full attention to everything we do. This would obviously limit our capacity to get things done. If we had to give every activity our full attention, it is doubtful that anyone would ever have invented the motor car or supermarkets. Our ability to routinize what we do frees up our minds for other challenges, and this has been a key factor in the evolution of the human species and in the way we now live our lives.

However, there is also a severe downside to our natural tendency to form habits: once we have learned to do certain things habitually and do them in a particular way, we find it very hard to change these behaviors. Even when we make a conscious decision to change, our non-conscious mind will take us back to our established habits.

Your non-conscious mind, which manages your habits, is fast and powerful. It manages your organs, blood pressure, and heart rate; it decides which of the things you see, hear, feel or taste should be put into memory and which should be discarded; it manages your automatic response to what is happening around you, for example, your stress response; and the list goes on. Scientists believe that the non-conscious mind drives more than 90 per cent of what we do.

Your non-conscious mind is also responsible for sorting through the quadrillion of memories stored in your mind to find those that are relevant to a situation you are facing. It connects memories and creates patterns – and it does all this regardless of whether you are awake or asleep.

Your non-conscious mind is far more powerful than any computer. This is why you are in safe hands when your non-conscious mind takes over when you are driving a car, and it's also why those who excel at certain sports are much more successful when they are on automatic pilot. It is not uncommon that somebody close to winning moves into conscious mode to think about the importance of the next round or the last few minutes of the game, only to find that they make a severe mistake and fail. This is because being in conscious mode meant they could not utilize the power of their non-conscious mind.

The conscious mind is slow and limited in capacity. In fact, you can't even use it to multitask. When you do more than one thing that demands your conscious attention at once, your mind will quickly switch back and forth between one task and the other. Unlike your non-conscious mind, which can do numerous things at once, your conscious mind can only just manage one stream of thought or activity at a time.

Your conscious mind is the part of the mind you use to decide to change your bad eating habits. The problem is that the nonconscious part of the mind that drives your bad eating habits is far more powerful than the part that drives your decision to change them. There is also another far more difficult barrier to accomplishing your goal of changing your habits: your conscious and non-conscious minds work in parallel, but they don't work together. In fact, any decision you make with your conscious mind (for example, 'I will lose 15 kg over the next three months') has absolutely no impact on your non-conscious mind. As I explained earlier, your non-conscious mind learns by repetition and not by instruction.

Conclusions

I will come back to how we might deal with this struggle between our conscious and non-conscious mind later. First, I want to summarize some of the key points:

- Human beings have a conscious and a non-conscious mind.
- While we tend to believe it is our conscious mind that decides what we do, it is largely the non-conscious mind that drives our behavior.
- Given the tremendous challenges we face in today's complex world, we can't give our full attention to everything we do; we need a non-conscious mind that can take over routine activities that don't require our full attention.
- Luckily for us, our non-conscious mind is faster and more powerful than our conscious mind. This allows us to delegate most of the routine things we do to our non-conscious mind, freeing up our conscious mind for the things we need or want to give attention to.

- When an unusual situation occurs, the non-conscious mind hands back the management to the conscious mind so we can give our full attention to the novel situation.
- Unfortunately, once our non-conscious mind is in charge of a behavior, it's difficult for us to change it. Our non-conscious mind doesn't follow the rational decisions we might make with our conscious mind; it learns through repetition – through establishing habits – rather than through instruction.

In summary, habits are learned behaviors, and learning is simply creating memories of 'how to do it' through repetitive behavior. Once you've had enough experience with a particular behavior, you can leave it to your non-conscious mind to take control. The non-conscious mind relies on the massive bank of memories it has built up by repeating this behavior again and again.

Habitual behaviors are great because they allow us to give our attention to other more rewarding matters or novel situations, while our non-conscious mind runs the activities in our life that are really just repeats. However, this useful habitualization strategy becomes a problem when we want to change the habits we have formed over time, such as our eating habits.

Goal Activation

Sometimes you trigger a need to eat without falling into habitual behavior. For example, you may feel a need to eat every time you walk past your fridge. This happens because in your mind the fridge and food are inextricably linked. Every time you take food out of the fridge or put food into it, you are strengthening this association. It is, therefore, no wonder that your fridge activates your desire to eat.

In neuroscience, we talk about goal activation. You have a natural goal to eat, and the fridge activates this goal and makes you feel like you really, really need to eat something *right then and there.*

There is sometimes only a fine line between a habit and an activated goal. For example, if, every time you walk past the fridge, you feel like eating but only occasionally do so, then we have a case of goal activation. If, however, you have a quick snack every time you walk past the fridge, then you have formed a habit (in this case, a bad eating habit).

For all practical purposes, it doesn't matter which of these it is, except that when you focus solely on habits, you tend to miss some important goal-activation triggers that may also be driving you towards eating more. For this reason, I have included a brief section on goal activation.

Both habits and goal activation are triggered by something. The trigger can be internal, such as your body running low on fuel and cueing a sensation of hunger; or they may be external, such as walking past the fridge, watching a food show on TV, sitting on the couch, feeling bored at work, preparing the school lunches for the children, cooking a meal, and so on. It is the external triggers that we are most interested in for the purposes of weight loss.

Some of the above-mentioned events and activities may trigger habits, while others may simply make you feel hungry without triggering a habitualized behavior, because you have not developed a habitual response to them; i.e., there is (not yet) a habitual behavior you automatically engage in after these activated goals. Rather, you might think, *Goodness, I AM hungry! I better get something to eat!'*, which is obviously a conscious thought rather than a non-conscious action (or habitualized action).

Clearly, you need to deal with both - habits and goal activation - to maximize your chances of success.

7

Turning bad habits into good habits

It is very likely that you have developed some bad eating habits over time. Maybe you automatically get out a bag of chips, an ice cream or some chocolate when you watch television at night, or maybe you take too many snack breaks during the day. Maybe you have just become used to consuming oversized portion sizes and feel hungry unless you get your usual quantity. Whatever bad habits you have learned, you now need to replace them with good habits.

To remind you of how habits work, let me go back one final time to the driving example: When you get into your car, the familiar environment triggers the driving behaviors. You don't have to consciously think, *I will now put the key into the ignition and fasten my seatbelt, and then step on the brake pedal while pushing the start button* (or whatever you have to do in your car). Your habitual mind simply takes over.

On the other hand, if you have ever rented an unfamiliar car or for that matter bought a new car, you have most likely experienced *alert triggers*. These include unfamiliar instruments or unfamiliar positioning of instruments on the dashboard or elsewhere. In these cases, you most likely had to give your conscious attention to starting the car and driving, at least until your mind became familiar enough with the car's particular features that your non-conscious mind could take over again.

In other words, there are three events that determine what happens:

- First, you must have 'trained' your mind by carrying out the same behavior many times before. You only develop a bad habit over time, by repeating the same behavior again and again. The number of times necessary will depend on how complex and variable the activity or its context is.

- Second, there have to be repeat triggers that tell your non-conscious mind to repeat a learned habit.

- Third, you may experience the occasional alert trigger that makes you aware of a bad habit you are just about to repeat or have already started to repeat.

As it is clearly too late to avoid developing bad eating habits, you have to focus on your repeat and alert triggers to make progress.

Let me also repeat once more that making a decision to change your bad eating habits won't have an impact on your behavior, because you will have made this decision with your conscious mind. This does not affect your non-conscious mind, which drives your bad habits.

Learn to make your old brain feel good!

This is the second Golden Rule, presented in the first part of this book. Hopefully you are already engaging in visualization on a regular basis. If not, now is the time to start! It will be almost impossible to break well established habits that deliver pleasure to your old brain unless you can deliver a positive experience through visualization.

Step 1: Eliminating repeat triggers

Your first strategy is to eliminate repeat triggers. It is unlikely that you can eliminate them all, but if you get rid of even just one repeat trigger, you can expect to get rid of one bad eating habit, which would certainly be a good start!

1. Identify your bad eating habits

If you usually have dessert after your dinner, a cigarette after a meal, or fall into a comfortable chair to watch television rather than read something useful when you get home from work, you are creating repeat triggers that tell your non-conscious mind it's time to get on with acting out the associated habitual behaviors. It's no surprise then that you find yourself automatically reaching for the ice cream, putting a cigarette in your mouth, or falling into 'your' chair as soon as you walk through your front door.

This is what you should do:

Over the next week, keep record of any bad eating habits you can identify. I recommend monitoring yourself for a whole week because your eating habits may be different on the weekend and during the week. Keep a notepad handy, and every time you find yourself eating, ask yourself if the drive to eat was due to a trigger that activated your bad eating habit (include also goal activation, i.e., drivers that make you think about eating food rather than leading to eating habits without giving it any thought).

Every evening, review your list and think about the day to ensure you haven't forgotten anything. Expect to feel even more like eating when you keep this list, because thinking all the time about your eating habits will remind your mind of the need and enjoyment associated with eating. But do persist. You have to start with a realistic assessment of what your bad eating habits are, otherwise you can hardly succeed in changing them.

2. Review each of these bad eating habits and identify the repeat triggers

Here are some triggers and their associated habitualized behaviors that cause overeating (these may trigger habits or activate your eating goal). Do any of these apply to you?

- ☐ starting to eat and then continuing automatically without even thinking about it
- ☐ taking a break from work and automatically reaching for food
- ☐ walking past the kitchen or fridge and stopping to get something to eat
- ☐ starting with a little snack and then keeping on going
- ☐ having a drink and then feeling like something to eat
- ☐ seeing others eat on television or in real life
- ☐ watching cooking shows or reading recipes
- ☐ walking past a fast-food restaurant
- ☐ feeling tired and eating to get more energy

All of these are examples of repeat triggers that lead to eating even when we're not hungry. It is important that you are very clear about the behaviors you want to change and that you identify the strongest triggers for these behaviors so you can find ways of weakening or even eliminating them.

This is what you should do:

For each eating habit, think about how it is triggered. The trigger is what happens immediately before you fall into the bad habit. For example, is watching television triggering snacking because you always snack when you watch TV?

Remember we also talked about 'goal activation'. This is a

trigger that leads you to *feel* like eating, although you have not (yet) developed a bad habit. You think about being hungry and feel like eating but you do not automatically, without any thought, start eating.

It is important for you to deal with both habitual eating and eating due to goal activation, so if you feel hungry every time you walk past the fridge or when you watch a cooking show on TV (goal activation stage), you need to make sure you deal with this situation before you develop bad eating habits.

It is important to give this some thought, because if you fail to identify the real triggers for your behavior, your ambition to change your habits will not be successful.

3. Try to find ways to eliminate the trigger.

The next, obvious, step is to eliminate as many of the triggers as possible. Be creative when you do this. Maybe you need to move the television or your comfortable armchair into the spare room until you have settled into a new routine. Perhaps you need to stop watching cooking programs or reading recipes for a while. Try to eliminate whatever it is that triggers the behavior you want to avoid.

4. List the actions you have decided to take

Don't try to change too much at the same time.

If possible, capitalize on any changes in your life or lifestyle (such as moving house or getting married, or when your children start school or leave home). It is often easier to break bad habits when your life starts to be quite different.

5. Work on developing good habits

While you can prevent yourself from falling into bad eating habits, this requires a massive amount of willpower and thus energy. The best way to avoid sapping these limited resources is to develop good eating habits. In other words, by repeating your good eating behavior over a long period of time, you start to develop good habits. This means the good behaviors occur without you having to put in effort or even think about it.

This is your opportunity to turn the force of habit into a positive effect. It will take a few weeks of disciplined repetition to achieve this, but once you have made it you will have eliminated a bad eating habit and adopted a good one for the long-term. It is a worthwhile investment that will lead to a happier and healthier life!

6. List the remaining repeat triggers and go to Step 2

Although you have a list of your repeat triggers and the actions you can take to eliminate or at least weaken them, it is likely that there are some you can't simply eliminate. This list of remaining repeat triggers is the focus of Step 2.

However, before you move on, you should give yourself time

to deal with the repeat triggers you *can* eliminate. Take the actions you have decided to take, see how well they work, improve or change your tactics, and, hopefully, eliminate at least some of your repeat triggers.

Then give yourself time to create good habits to replace the old, bad habits.

Don't move on to the next set of actions too quickly. It takes time for your brain to change the way it works. You can't rush it. Don't forget that some of your habits may have taken many years to establish themselves; you can't expect to change them over night.

The following are some signs that you are ready to move on to Strategy 2:

- you very rarely fall back into the old habit you are trying to eliminate;
- you don't feel any pressure or frustration with respect to this old eating habit;
- you experience a feeling of success because you were able to make a significant dent into your bad habits;
- you are relaxed and confident that you have found a way to effectively deal with the eating habit you are targeting.
  When you are ready move on to Step 2.

Step 2: Develop alert triggers that make you aware of bad eating habits before you start eating...

7. Create Alert Triggers

You need to eliminate repeat triggers whenever possible, but sometimes there is no way you can. For example, when you care for a family, you can't just keep less food at home – after all, your children and partner will need to be looked after. But you can establish alert triggers that bring your habitual behavior into your conscious thought. This means that you don't look back and think, *I've done it again – last night I....* Instead, you become consciously involved at the very time the habitual behavior you are trying to avoid begins to manifest itself.

Alert triggers are events that are not part of the normal routine. In fact, sometimes removing a repeat trigger in itself creates an alert trigger. For example, keeping less food in the fridge makes it less likely for you to routinely go to the fridge and grab some food while also reminding you (when you see the near-empty fridge) of your decision to change your eating habits. Your conscious mind will come into play and you will think, *That's right! I did that to help me stop my habitual eating!*

Depending on what habit you are trying to change, you may find it effective to

- send yourself reminders (e.g., delayed email delivery or

mobile phone alerts);

- ask friends or family to remind you of your resolution;

- change the environment (shift the furniture, use rooms differently, eat in the backyard or on the balcony...);

- change your plates and glasses to smaller sized ones (unless you drink water - drinking plenty of water is OK);

- put notes to yourself on the fridge/your table/your desk;

- book a wake-up call with a specific message;

- put a note on your dog's collar reminding you to take her for a walk.

There are endless possibilities. Experiment to find what works for you. It is also possible that an alert trigger will work initially but that when you get used to it (that is, when you habitualize the trigger) it won't have as much impact anymore and you will need to replace it with a new alert trigger.

Review the list of repeat triggers you have been unable to eliminate and consider each one carefully for better ways to manage it. Try to find ways of alerting your conscious mind *before* you fall into the bad eating habit; i.e., move eating from a non-conscious habit to a conscious decision.

8. Find ways of dealing with your need to eat once you have become aware of it

Allow yourself to make trade-off decisions

While this is, strictly speaking, a way to make the old

behavior less attractive, it represents a very different approach.

Rather than try to simply 'ban' the behavior you want to change, allow yourself to engage in old habits – but only when you 'pay' a price for doing so. In other words, you offer yourself two options: don't engage in old habits, or do engage but pay a penalty.

To illustrate this strategy, let's assume you decide that the payment to be made for eating when you shouldn't comprises of sit-ups. Note that all payments need to be made up-front. This is a very important point because if you delay the payment, you are likely to conveniently find no time to pay it later. Having decided on the price, you could stick a note on the fridge door outlining the trade-off – something like *'1 snack = 20 sit-ups.'*

This approach is useful for two reasons: first, it forces you to make a conscious decision. Second, it treats you like an adult. Rather than saying 'don't do this,' like you might to a child who can't yet understand reason, you are giving yourself two options to choose from.

It is, however, important that you change the price in light of your behavior.

If you decide that you won't have the snack to avoid the 20 sit-ups, you can leave the number of sit-ups the same for next time, but if you find yourself making the trade-off easily (i.e., doing the 20 sit-ups to get the snack), then you need to increase the price – perhaps to 25 sit-ups – for next time. Eventually you will find the level where you would rather forego the snack than do the sit-ups.

Naturally, simply ignoring the trade-off rule and having the snack without paying for it would represent a step back. Try to avoid falling into the trap of ignoring the trade-off (or any other decision you may have made to eliminate or reduce bad habits), and be aware that you are more likely to do this when you are feeling weak.

Avoid weakening your conscious mind

It is very easy to fall back into old habits when you are tired or have had too much to drink. When your conscious mind is weakened, your non-conscious mind takes over. Again, this is a great mechanism for fighting for survival in a hostile environment, but in your world it simply means that you will rapidly fall back into your bad old habits.

I understand that it is not always possible to avoid tiredness, but you can put a greater emphasis on rest and try to get a little extra rest here and there. Alcohol is another problem because it clouds your judgment and may also make you feel good or even invincible. In your artificially 'relaxed' state you are more likely to reject the change you are trying to make and engage in the old behavior – if you are able to think about your trade-off at all.

It is important to be aware that weakening your conscious mind may take you back to old habits and that sometimes this is difficult to avoid. If you can avoid it, do so. If you can't, focus on the other strategies you can employ.

8

Willpower is a limited resource

Back to pre-historic times: Arfast's Story

Arfast is part of a tribe lead by Gronet, the strongest of the men. They hunt together, each giving their best, as they are always hungry. But when it comes to sharing food, there are always fights. In fact, it's only a matter of time before Arfast's drive to get a bigger share of the food will annoy Gronet – and that's likely to be the last we hear of Arfast...

Here is your question: *What would you ideally want Arfast's brain to do to help him survive?*

I have to admit, this is a bit of a misleading question: Arfast's brain won't be able to develop quickly enough to escape his fate. My question should be, what capabilities do you feel the brain has to develop to help Arfast's progeny avoid such a fate in the future?

We want the brain to develop the ability to control our behavior, to understand social norms and other norms, and to be able to follow them for our own benefit. In fact, this is exactly what the brain did. Some 100,000 years ago, we developed the frontal lobes (the part of the brain behind your forehead). The frontal lobes give us the ability to think rationally about the consequences of our actions. Because humans are a social species, much of the restraint we need to exercise is social in nature.

Some anthropologists believe that the smartest non-human primates can project about twenty minutes into the future, which is long enough to let the strongest male eat first without interference. After 20 minutes, their willpower is exhausted and they just get on with fighting for food.

Being able to hold out for 20 minutes may be sufficient for an animal to survive by being able to hold off fighting for a chunk of meat, but it is not going to be sufficient when it comes to resisting food when you are attempting to change your eating habits.

What is willpower?

According to *Wikipedia*, willpower is

- **Self-discipline**: training and control of oneself and one's conduct, usually for personal improvement
- **Self-control**: the ability of a person to exert his/her will over the inhibitions of their body or self.

Obviously, then, willpower is something you need if you wish to change your eating behavior.

Having a high degree of willpower changes one's life

In their book *Willpower: Rediscovering the Greatest Human Strength*, Roy F. Baumeister and John Tierney report that children who showed the most willpower at age four went on to get better grades and test scores later in their lives.[5] This statement is based on an early-childhood willpower test in which children were asked to resist the urge to immediately eat a marshmallow.

Years later, the researchers followed up with the children who had participated in the research program and who had since entered adulthood. They then compared the lives of the high- and low-willpower group.

The research results showed that children with high willpower grew up to become more popular with their peers and their teachers and earned higher salaries. They also had a lower body-mass index; i.e. their willpower seemed to have allowed them to avoid putting on as much weight as the low-willpower group. They were also less likely to report having had problems with drug abuse.

These findings were confirmed by a study of Asian-Americans who placed great importance on teaching their children to develop self-discipline rather than on developing

---

[5] Roy F Baumeister and John Tierney, *Willpower: Rediscovering the Greatest Human Strength*, The Penguin Press, NY 2011, pp 194–195

high self-esteem, which was the more fashionable approach in the United States late last century. Baumeister and Tierney reported that a two-year-old Chinese child is expected to have levels of impulse control that correspond roughly to what American children are expected to have at age three or four.

They note that

Asian-Americans make up only 4% of the US population but account for a quarter of the student body at elite universities like Stanford, Columbia and Cornell. They're more likely to get a college degree than any other ethnic group, and they go on the earn salaries that are 25% above the American norm. Elite jobs like physicians, scientists, and accountants require a high IQ. For Americans the average IQ for these elite professionals is 110, but Chinese-Americans get the same jobs with an average IQ of only 102. But the story does not end there. Chinese-Americans have higher rates of actually getting into those jobs, meaning that a Chinese-American with an IQ above 103 is more likely to get an elite job than an American with an IQ above 110.

These and other studies clearly show that willpower is a greater asset than intelligence when it comes to achievement. Clearly, you have to have some intelligence, but strong willpower with an average IQ is likely to get you further than a high IQ and little willpower.

Willpower depletion

You don't only get physically tired from being busy all day; your willpower also gets 'tired' when you overuse it. Willpower is a limited resource, which means that you eventually run out of it. Given that it is a limited resource, we need to understand first what uses our willpower up and, second, how to replenish it.

The problem is that you use willpower not only when you are resisting a temptation but also when you are making a decision. Kelly McGonical reports on a study where people were asked how many food-related decisions they made in one day.[6] Before you read on, what's your best guess? How many food decisions do you think you might make during a typical day?

In the McGonical study, the average guess among the participants was 14, but when these people carefully kept track of their decisions, the true average turned out to be 227. And these are just decisions related to food (which includes preparing a shopping list, selecting food in the grocery store, cooking or preparing food, eating food, serving food, preparing food for school lunches, preserving food, etc.).

Given that the average person most likely makes somewhere around 227 decisions just related to food, imagine how many

---

[6] McGonical Kelly, *The Willpower Instinct: How Self-Control Works, Why It Matters and What You Can Do to Get More of It*, New York 2012, p.21

decisions you would make in total per day? Think about all the other decisions you make – from which clothes to wear to what to do with your leisure time. Consider all the decisions you might make at work or at home, when meeting with friends or visiting relatives, when having guests or when simply deciding what to watch on television in the evening.

If you are responsible for a family – and in particular for younger children – there are a whole host of additional decisions to be made every day. And every one of these decisions drains you of a little bit of willpower.

You may find the idea that making decisions depletes your willpower hard to believe, but there are numerous studies that confirm this. For example, a research study in a shopping center showed that shoppers who had already made plenty of decisions in various stores had less willpower than those who just started out on their shopping expedition. Their willpower was measured by how long it took them to give up when asked to carry out some simple arithmetic problems.

Willpower depletion is sometimes used to make sales. For example, it has been demonstrated that a car dealer can boost the revenue generated by a sale by taking a car buyer through low-cost accessory and customization options first, leaving the higher margin options until later when the customer's willpower has been depleted.

In the context of weight loss, depletion of willpower might

mean that by the end of the day you simply do not have enough willpower left to stick to your eating plans.

Glucose is your willpower fuel

Wikipedia tells us that the name 'glucose' comes from the Greek word *'glukus'*, meaning 'sweet'. The suffix '-*ose'* denotes a sugar. Glucose, also known as D-glucose, dextrose or grape sugar, is a simple sugar and an important carbohydrate in biology.

Glucose fuels your willpower. If you experience a lack of glucose, you will find that your willpower drains away. This creates a particularly difficult catch-22 situation: when you exercise self-control, your body uses up glucose, which makes you feel like eating something sweet. To be able to exercise self-control and stick with your decision to eat less, you need more glucose, but eating something sugary most likely will derail your plans.

As if this is not difficult enough, women also have to fight the need for more glucose during menstruation. Baumeister explains that during the

> ... *premenstrual part of the cycle, which is called the luteal phase, the female body starts channeling a high amount of its energy to the ovaries and to related activities, like producing extra quantities of female hormones. As more energy and glucose are diverted to the reproductive system, there's less*

available for the rest of the body, which responds by craving more food. Chocolate and other sweets are immediately appealing because they provide instant glucose, but any kind of food can help, which is why women report more food cravings and tend to eat more. One study found that the average woman eats about 810 calories at lunch during this time, which is about 170 calories more than what she eats at lunch during the rest of the month.[7]

Lack of sleep and alcohol

Golden Rule No3 referred to sleep and alcohol. As your willpower is affected by both I decided to add to the earlier discussion.

Glucose is the main form of energy that fuels your willpower. When you are overtired, your cells have trouble absorbing glucose from the bloodstream. You experience a feeling of exhaustion and start to crave sweet food or caffeine because your body is desperate for energy. Even if you give in and indulge in sweet foods, you will most likely find that the impact is not that great, simply because your cells are struggling to absorb the glucose you have pumped too quickly into your bloodstream.

The first challenge is therefore to get enough sleep and,

---

[7] *Roy F Baumeister and John Tierney, ibid. pp 53–54*

whenever possible, to have a nap when you feel tired. When you sleep, you are no longer depleting your glucose level through activities such as making decisions or exercising self-control. I am sure you have observed in the past that when you are tired, your self-control is much lower; you are more likely to cave in and deviate from your weight loss journey.

Another factor that causes a lack of self-control is alcohol. When you drink, you start to lose your ability to monitor your own behavior and this eventually leads to a loss of self-control. In this state, it is natural to simply eat whatever you feel like – and lots of it!

You will find it easier to reach and maintain a Happy Weight if you manage your willpower effectively, i.e., by avoiding rapid depletion, refueling your willpower regularly and training your willpower to make it stronger.

9

Boosting your willpower

Step 1: Work out when your willpower is weak

The first step is to identify any patterns: does your willpower seem reduced at certain times of the day, on certain occasions, in certain places, or when particular people are with you, etc.?

Over the next week, keep record of any occasions during the day when you feel your willpower has let you down. Keep a notepad handy and every time you find your willpower to be weak, write down the situation and what happened.

Every evening, review your list and think about the day to see if you have forgotten something.

Step 2: Work out WHY your willpower is weak on these occasions.

Is it because you have tried really hard to change your bad eating habits, or because you had to make too many decisions earlier in the day, or because you are overtired or consumed alcohol, or because you are emotionally drained or are going through the luteal phase of your menstrual cycle, etc.?

Step 3: Identify any ways you can fix the problem

For example, have more sleep, drink less, or try to make fewer decisions. Make a list of what you could do to increase your willpower and note when you will take action, and then try to stick with it...

Step 4: Train your willpower to make it stronger

There are likely to be remaining willpower issues you can't address directly, as suggested in the previous step. Rather, you have to train your willpower so that you have more of it and so that, even with the normal depletion, there is more left over when you end up in situations that make it difficult to stick with your new eating habits.

If you exercise your brain in the same way again and again, it will allocate more neurons to the task. For example, brain scans of London taxi drivers showed that they have a larger area allocated to undertaking spatial tasks, because they often use this part of the brain when they work out the best route to take to get from A to B.

The same allocation of neurons occurs when any mental activity is regularly engaged. And, as willpower is a mental activity, this also applies to the development of willpower. In other words, by using your willpower often you can strengthen it in the same way taxi drivers strengthen their spatial abilities. Here are some ways of doing that:

You can train your willpower by simply making a commitment to making a change in your life. The good news is that your goal does not have to be something as difficult as weight loss. You can train your willpower by making an easier change – at least to start with. McGonical suggests selecting your challenge from one of the following:[8]

- Strengthen 'I Won't" Power – Commit to not swearing, to not crossing your legs when you sit, or to using your non-dominant hand for a daily task such as eating or operating doors.

- Strengthen 'I Will' Power – Commit to doing something every day (not something you already do) just for the practice of building a habit and not making excuses. It could be anything from calling your mother to meditating for five minutes....

- Strengthen *Self-Monitoring* – Formally keep track of something you don't usually pay close attention to. This could be your spending, what you eat, or how much time you spend online or watching TV.

Research has shown that exercising willpower increases people's stamina, allowing them to hold out against temptations even when their mental resources have been depleted.

---

[8] McGonical Kelly, *The Willpower Instinct: How Self-Control Works, Why It Matters and What You Can Do to Get More of It*, New York 2012, p. 68

For example, participants who practiced exercising their willpower in a study were able to advance toward their goals. Those in the fitness program got fitter, those working on study discipline got more schoolwork done, and those in the money management program saved more money.

But – and here is a truly pleasant surprise – the participants also got better at advancing at their other personal goals. In other words, they had strengthened their willpower.

Step 5: Turn your new behaviour into a habit

Research has shown that people with high self-control use their self-control to develop good habits. By repeating the desirable behavior again and again, they eventually habitualize it, and once that has happened they don't need to spend any of their limited willpower resources on making sure they avoid their bad habits. In other words, once you have used your willpower to develop good eating habits, such as smaller portion sizes or eating the right foods, you will no longer need to use willpower to continue the habit.

To me, this is the most exciting aspect of losing weight: you do have to make an effort to make it happen initially, but if you stick with good eating habits for long enough, these good habits will stay with you for life – without you having to continually use your willpower to maintain your weight.

The development of good habits is the ultimate

achievement. This doesn't just apply to weight loss or, more importantly, to maintaining your weight over time.

Baumeister uses academics to illustrate this point: they have to publish to progress in their careers. Research showed that academics who developed the habit of writing just a few pages (even just a page a day) did well and often got tenure, while those who wrote only occasionally and put out huge amounts in short periods of time typically got stuck in their careers as they could not spark these writing binges often enough.[9] The conclusion: regular habits outperform the occasional big effort!

Finally, here are some strategies you can employ should all else fail:

To change, decide that you will never change...

I have come across some interesting research that suggests that one of the main reasons people procrastinate is because they feel they can start tomorrow. For some reason, we always expect that tomorrow we will be able to do what we feel unable or unwilling to do today. And given that we start tomorrow we are only delaying the benefits that the changed behavior brings by one day. Of course, the next day we may feel that the day after is a better day to start, and so on....

Behavioral economist Howard Rachlin proposed an

---

[9] Roy F Baumeister and John Tierney, ibid., p. 159

interesting approach to overcoming the problem of always starting a change tomorrow. Simply make a commitment to eat the *same* amount of food every day from now on. This means that every piece of cake, dob of ice cream, huge serve of potato mash and greasy hamburgers you have today you will eat every day from today onwards.

This means that you can't pretend any longer that tomorrow will be different. Because the plan is to repeat your behavior, every meal or snack becomes not just one you have today, but one you will have tomorrow, and the day after that, and the day after that. This adds new weight to overeating and makes it much harder to deny the lifestyle and health consequences of eating excessively.[10]

Defer the reward eating offers, just a little

This is also called the postponed-pleasure ploy: tell yourself that you can have a desert later if you still want it. Meanwhile, eat something else. The body feels a desire for sweet foods, but that is only because it is a familiar and effective way to restore energy. Healthy foods will also provide the energy it needs.

Remember also that being in a depleted state makes you feel everything more intensely than usual. Desires and cravings are exceptionally intense to the depleted mind. Dieting is a frequent drain on your willpower, and so you will frequently fall into a depleted state.

Make a pre-commitment

You can sign a commitment contract with StickK.com along with a penalty that will be imposed automatically if you don't reach it. You can monitor yourself or nominate a referee to report on your success or failure. The penalty may simply be a round of emails from stickK.com to your designated list of supporters, or you can also make it financially costly by setting up an automatic payment from your credit card to charity.

People who draw up a contract without a financial penalty or a referee succeed only 35 per cent of the time, whereas the ones with a penalty and a referee succeed nearly 80 per cent of the time. Likewise, those who risk more than $100 do better than those who risk less than twenty dollars.

Reward often

Online games became essentially the largest experiment ever conducted into motivational strategies. By getting instant feedback from millions of on-line players, the game designers learned precisely which incentives work: namely, a mix of frequent small prizes with occasional big prizes. Even when

---

[10] McGonical Kelly, *The Willpower Instinct: How Self-Control Works, Why It*

players lose battles or make mistakes or cause their avatars to die, they remain motivated because of the emphasis on rewards rather than punishment. Instead of feeling they have failed, the players think that they just haven't succeeded yet.

The final chapter of this book encourages you to celebrate achievements – even small ones – often. It is important to stay positive, and one way of achieving this is to celebrate.

10

Stress is a major cause of weight gains...

Stories from another time: Hagar's Story

Hagar is one of your distant ancestors who lived a few hundred thousand years ago. For Hagar and his tribe to survive, he must hunt. There is a good chance that rather than kill an animal, he will be killed himself; nevertheless, without hunting, there is no food, an even more certain death – for him and his tribe.

Hagar doesn't know this, of course. His brain is not yet far enough developed to understand cause and effect, or to consider the future consequences of today's actions and events. What he does know is that he is hungry, and his instinct tells him that he needs to get a kill today.

As he carefully sneaks along, club in hand, there is a sudden movement in the bushes. He is hoping for an easy kill. But a saber-toothed tiger emerges – four times his weight, and ten times as fast as he is. Maybe even a hundred times faster, given that Hagar's body is run down from lack of food.

Now it is truly kill or be killed. His fingers close around the club so tightly his knuckles nearly burst. The moment of truth has arrived...

Sorry, end of story! Now it's your turn: *What would you want Hagar's brain to do in this situation to help him to survive?*

Take a couple of minutes to put together your wish list for Hagar's brain. Then read on.

Here is what his brain *will* do for him: It will produce adrenalin and cortisol. The adrenalin will give him more energy and strength, and the cortisol will encourage his body to create fat cells.

Energy and strength will increase Hagar's chances of killing and lower the chances of him being killed. Or, if he simply ends up running as fast as he can, it will help him run faster for longer and thus increase his chances of survival. He won't be able to outrun a saber-toothed tiger, but if he can outrun one of his hunting partners he may be all right.

If he kills the tiger and eats the meat, the additional fat cells will make it possible for him to store more food, allowing him to survive for a longer period before his next kill.

Is this more or less what you put on your wish list? Or is it even *more* than you asked for?

I think it is absolutely marvelous that the brain has

developed such a great response to life-threatening situations. However, although the brain works to increase our chances of staying alive in a hostile environment, this doesn't necessarily help us in the environment we live in today. After all, how useful is a stress response that encourages your body to produce more fat cells and your mind to eat lots of comfort food?

Fast forward to today...

In her 2010 book *The Willpower Instinct*, Kelly McGonical refers to a 2010 national survey by the American Psychological Association that shows that 75 per cent of people in the United States experience high levels of stress.[11] There is hardly anyone these days who doesn't live in (and perhaps also work in) a stressful environment.

Not surprisingly, Americans reported indulging in unhealthy foods more often to cope with the stress in their lives, and smokers reported smoking more cigarettes and giving up attempts to quit.

Stress is something that has served humans very well for thousands of years. In the case of Hagar and the saber-toothed tiger, he experienced acute stress when facing the tiger. His brain immediately released chemicals that do the following:

---

[11] McGonical Kelly, *The Willpower Instinct: How Self-Control Works, Why It Matters and What You Can Do to Get More of It*, New York 2012, p.52-53

- deliver a short-term boost in strength and energy, enabling him to run faster or to have a better chance of killing the saber-toothed tiger
- generate fat cells, allowing him to store more food (if he succeeded in making the kill and eating the meat) and thus remain safer for longer.

As soon as the stress is over (which would happen for Hagar when he either escaped or defeated the saber-toothed tiger), the brain goes back to normal. Most likely, situations like Hagar found himself in would not have lasted longer than a few minutes. The stress our forebears experienced was *acute*, i.e., generated by an event or situation that was intense but played out over a brief period of time.

And that's where the problem lies: today, stress is an on-going feature of many people's life. Difficult financial situations, constant traffic jams, unreliable public transport, worrisome children, noisy neighbors, workplace stress or whatever else it may be is *chronic*, as it persists over long periods of time.

This means that your brain is actively producing chemicals that prepare you for fight or flight when in fact your best course of action would be to ignore the stress, step back, review the situation, and then make a decision on what (if anything) can be done.

Of course, it is useful to have a strong stress response when facing a crocodile or a bear in the wild, but these dangers were more common in the world of our distant ancestors rather than the world we live in today.

I am sure that the human brain will work quite differently in a few million years (if the human species survives that long), but today we must each deal with a brain that is designed for the kind of hostile environment we no longer live in. The fight-or-flight response that has served humankind well for thousands of years is no longer useful. Today's stress generators tend to be around us regularly, if not permanently, resulting in chronic stress.

This means that stress is simply making our lot worse rather than preparing us to respond effectively to potentially life-threatening challenges. Given that our built-in response to chronic stress is damaging rather than useful, we need to change this response.

This poses an interesting challenge because the stress response is managed by our non-conscious mind; we can't reduce or eliminate stress by simply deciding to do so. We need to find a way to use the processes that reside in our non-conscious mind to our advantage; i.e., we need to short-circuit our hard-wired stress responses. But before we can do that, we need a better understanding of how stress works.

Symptoms of stress

The purpose of this chapter is not to provide you with an overview on stress symptoms. If you want to learn more about stress and related symptoms, I suggest you visit the Mayo Clinic website (www.mayoclinic.com), which is one of the most authoritative medical websites in the world.

All I will do here is repeat some of the symptoms the Mayo Clinic lists on its website:

... if your mind and body are constantly on edge because of excessive stress in your life, you may face serious health problems. That's because your body's 'fight-or-flight' reaction is constantly on.

Adrenalin increases your heart rate, elevates your blood pressure and boosts energy supplies. Cortisol, the primary stress hormone, increases sugars (glucose) in the bloodstream....

Cortisol also curbs functions that would be nonessential or detrimental in a fight-or-flight situation. It alters immune system responses and suppresses the digestive system, the reproductive system and growth processes. This complex natural system also communicates with regions of your brain that control mood, motivation and fear.

The resulting effects of stress on...

- *your body* include headaches, back pain, chest pain, heart disease, obesity, high blood pressure, sleep problems and stomach upsets.

- *your thoughts and feelings* include anxiety, restlessness, worrying, irritability, lack of focus, forgetfulness, and anger.
- *your behavior* include overeating, angry outbursts, drug- or alcohol-abuse, relationship conflicts and social withdrawal.

Of particular concern is the fact that decisions made under stress are not likely to be good decisions. Stress may prevent you from making decisions at all, or it may lead you to make a decision when you are unable to clearly focus on the issues or think through the consequences of your decisions. This may lead to actions you later regret, which is likely to increase your level of stress even further.

Add to this the damage stress can cause to your relationships with family, friends, work colleagues and others, as well as the impact stress can have on the atmosphere at home or at work, on your well-being, career and general standing within your community or company, and it is clear that ensuring you don't become a victim of stress is of vital importance.

But let me focus on our main concern in this book: stress is a major cause of weight gain! Not many people fully appreciate how much stress contributes to gaining weight.

Stress is causing overeating

Here is an unfortunately common chain of events that leads to weight gain:

1. You are stressed.
2. When stressed, you resort to 'comfort food', which is typically unhealthy or high-kilojoule food.
3. When you eat the comfort food, you feel better.
4. But the feeling doesn't last. The stress returns. And you need more comfort food....

If you have ever experienced a 'comfort food occasion', you are just a normal person living in our stressful times. But let's explore this more fully. Let's first have a look at the impact of *acute* stress:

Stress causes your brain – more precisely, the hypothalamus – to produce CRF (corticotrophin-releasing factor). This in turn stimulates your adrenal gland to produce large amounts of hormones – namely, adrenal corticosteroids, including cortisol.

It does not matter if you don't remember the medical terms; the main point is that these hormones dampen down your immune system, increase alertness and quicken your heart rate. They get you into the best possible state to deal with an acute stress situation: alert and bristling with energy. They also help your liver to convert fat into energy, and they signal to your body to accumulate fat cells in the abdomen.

All of this would have been extremely useful to our forebears when they were hunting. The rush would have increased their likelihood of success, and the fat cells would have allowed them to store more food. After all, they couldn't just drop into a 7-Eleven or fast-food outlet to satisfy their appetite on the way home.

With acute stress, there is no obesity problem: the impact is short term and the brain stops producing CRF when the danger (the acute stress) is over. The following diagram shows this process of what happens when you experience acute stress.

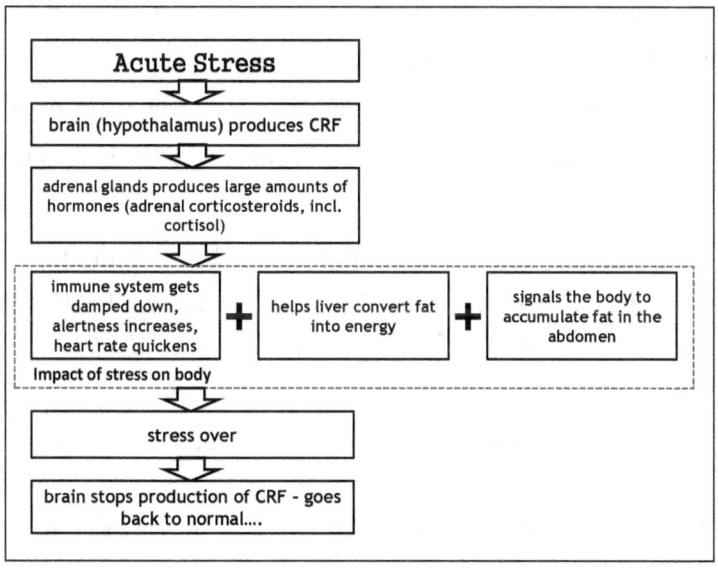

Now let's turn our attention to chronic stress. What

happens when you are exposed to stress over long periods of time? [12, 13]

The initial process is pretty much the same as with acute stress. This should not come as a surprise, as we are talking about a general stress response. Your brain doesn't assess stress, classify it and then pick the appropriate response depending on what sort of stress it might be. The difference is that with chronic stress, the stress impulse doesn't go away. As the fat cells are generated, you feel like eating foods that are high in fat and carbohydrates; i.e., you crave so-called comfort foods.

The interesting and very important point is that the consumption of these foods *does* in fact lead to a reduction in the stress you are experiencing. It signals to the brain that things are now under control, and, as a result, the brain stops producing CRF. In other words, comfort foods really do help us to feel better.

However, this relief is short-lived. Soon your stress experience returns to 'normal' – that is, to the level you

---

[12] Sources: Dallman, Mary F et al., *Chronic Stress and Obesity: A New View of "Comfort Food'*, in Proceedings of the National Academy of Sciences, Sep 30, 2003, Vol 100, no 20, pp. 11696ff.

[13] Goodman Elizabeth and Robert C Whitaker, *A Prospective Study of the Role of Depression in the Development and Persistence of Adolescent Obesity'*, in Pediatrics, Vol 109, No 3, September 2002, pp. 497 ff.; Sarah Mustillo et al, *Obesity and Psychiatric Disorder: Developmental Trajectories*, in Pediatrics, Vol 111, No 4, April 2003, pp. 851 ff.

experienced before you indulged in comfort food. You go through another cycle, and another, and another after that, and so on. And as you struggle through all this stress, you put on weight.

The following diagram illustrates this process.

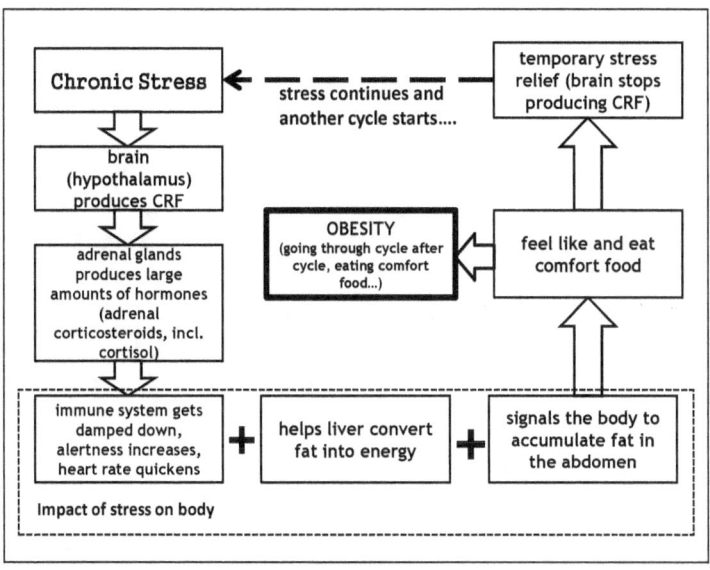

Chronic stress causes you to put on weight by causing the production of cortisol, which encourages the production of fat cells and the eating of comfort foods. Worse, once they have been produced, fat cells want to be fed – and they are very hard to shed.

Research has also shown that depression is a cause of

obesity rather than a consequence. Depressed people who are not overweight at the onset of their depression have a twofold increase in the risk of becoming obese.

11

Living without stress

If you suffer from stress, you will find it difficult to make significant changes to your life because stress will derail you again and again, lead you to eat large quantities of comfort food, sap your willpower, tire you out and make your life a misery. For this reason, I feel you should make every effort to eliminate stress from your life.

However, if you don't suffer from stress, then skip this chapter as it will be of no interest to you.

1   Understanding Stress

The problem with stress is that it draws you into a downward spiral. Something triggers it and, once you are stressed, you become irritated by other factors that may not themselves have caused stress but seem unbearable when you are already in a stressed state.

For example, when you are facing some financial difficulty, stress starts to build. Because you are tense and worried, you may become excessively annoyed by noises that in less-stressful times you would simply have ignored. In your already stressed state, you become even more stressed due to this noise irritation.

With your stress levels reaching a dangerous high, you may end up in an argument with your partner or one of your colleagues about, well, nothing really; or you may send a terse email to someone or take out your stress on the children or pets. Once done, you regret your actions, and this increases your stress further. And so you go further and further down the stress spiral.

The first and most important step is to avoid this spiral in the first place.

The only way you can do this is to step out of the stressful situation you are in – that is, to break the connection between yourself and how you feel. You need to disengage emotionally by stepping back and taking a look at how you feel and what is happening to you.

Stepping back gets harder and harder the more stressed you get and the longer the stress continues, so the first step is to understand how this spiral starts; namely, by identifying what particular trigger points cause feelings of stress to surface.

It makes good sense to write these trigger points down. Even just the process of observing what is happening to you and recording the stressors will allow you to become somewhat detached from the stressful event.

Sometimes triggers are very easy to identify, for example,

they may be checking your latest bank statement or listening to the children screaming for hours on end. At other times the triggers may not be so obvious. You may feel stressed without being quite sure as to what is causing it. In these instances, it is particularly useful to record potential triggers and then to adapt and refine your list every time that type of stress occurs.

The second step is to be aware of how you feel about the stressful event. Do you experience fear, uncertainty, confusion, annoyance? Do negative attitudes or opinions start to bubble up in your mind? Would you rather be somewhere else or with somebody else?

The third step is to become aware of how you react to the stress. Do you let your temper fly? Do you overeat? Do you experience physical pain, such as headaches? Do you feel depressed?

Again, observing how you feel allows you to detach yourself.

2 Managing Stress

Once you are already stressed, you may find it difficult to go through the steps outlined above. It may occur to you that you should, but in your stressed state of mind you may decide that this is all nonsense anyway, that you have no time, or that you will be able to deal with it without going through all this.

It is therefore important that you have a circuit breaker you can trigger in your mind. Creating a circuit breaker is very simple – imagine something really positive, meaningful and calming. However, this task relies on you taking it seriously and repeating it until the response becomes almost automatic.

Call up your chosen image in your mind **as soon as you feel even the slightest build-up of stress**. Your visualization will provide you with a small oasis of calm – just enough to break the stress circuit.

I read some time back in a *Harvard Business Review* article (I can't recall the title or authors, I'm afraid) that even just training your mind to call up a picture of something pleasant and engaging can be enough to break the circuit. This makes sense, as the stress you are experiencing is occurring only in your mind.

It is important to note that calling up this image *will not eliminate the stressful situation*. It won't make it go away. You will feel stressed again before too long. But once you can call up this picture without effort – once it becomes an almost automatic reaction to stress – you will find that it helps you to avoid going down the stress spiral.

The sequence for creating this circuit breaker is as follows:

- As soon as you feel any stress at all, call up your positive image (it should always be the same image so you can condition your mind).
- You will feel temporary relief as your mind experiences positive feelings. Take this opportunity to address the three

questions raised earlier:

○ What is triggering the stress you experienced?

○ What did you feel as a result of this stress?

○ How did you react to the stress (or, hopefully, how would you have reacted had you not called up the positive image in your mind)?

3   Eliminating Stress

You will feel a great burden lifted off your shoulders once you have mastered the art of managing stress. There are, of course, serious life events that will lead to stress, no matter how prepared you are. These include negative life-changing events such as the death of someone close, a serious accident, divorce, or losing your job.

However, most of the chronic stress we experience does not fall into the serious life events category (although a poor response to chronic stress may eventually lead to a life-changing event). Ultimately, I believe you should strive to *eliminate* the chronic stress that results from situations that may be unfortunate but are by no means unusual.

The problem is that when you are stressed, you will find it much more difficult to deal with these situations. Breaking the stress circuit is great – at least you won't get dragged down into the depths of negative feelings or suffer the physical reactions that stress can cause. But what if you could avoid experiencing negative stress all together?

I say 'negative' stress because positive stress can be a great contributor to success. Positive stress, also called eustress, allows you to use the chemicals your brain is producing in response to stress in a constructive way. Importantly, the event lasts for a limited time – that is, you do not experience chronic stress.

Let's suppose there is an important event you are responsible for, like a wedding or a major family reunion, or perhaps you have to attend a job interview. In such a situation, it may be helpful to have the extra energy and drive that stress hormones can give you. Then, after a short period, it's all over, and your mind will return to normal – although you may feel a bit tired from the effort.

This is all fine. What we are trying to avoid is the negative impact that *chronic* stress can cause.

I was lucky enough to learn, early in my work life, a simple technique that allowed me to do just that. I had moved from the University of Vienna to an Australian university but had maintained a relationship with Austria's preeminent executive training center, Hernstein. I regularly flew back to Austria to lead executive programs. On one of these occasions, an invitation was issued by another seminar leader who happened to be at Hernstein at the same time, Professor Jagdish Parikh.

He invited other seminar leaders to attend an early, pre-breakfast session to learn more about 'Managing the Self' (the title of his seminar and also, later, a book authored by Prof. Parikh).

In this session, I learned a very simple relaxation technique:

- sit in a chair that gives you great back support; keep your back straight and your head upright; put your feet flat on the ground and rest your hands on your thighs; do not let your left and right hand legs or hands touch (simply leave a little space between your knees and feet).

- close your eyes

- focus your attention on the top of your head and relax any tense muscles you can feel there

- go down your face and relax any tense muscles you can feel there

- go down the back of your head to your neck and relax any tense muscles you can feel there

- go down your neck to your shoulders and relax any tense muscles in your shoulders

- go down your chest and relax any tense muscles

- go down your stomach and relax any tense muscles you can feel there

- go back to your shoulders and this time go down your back and relax any tense muscles you can feel there

- go down your bottom and relax any tense muscles you can feel there

- go down your thighs and relax any tense muscles
- go down your legs and relax any tense muscles you can feel there
- go down your feet and relax any tense muscles
- go down your toes and relax any tense muscles you can feel there
- now sit still and enjoy how relaxed you are
- take your time and when you are ready open your eyes.

If you are really tensed up you may want to run through this sequence twice rather than just once. And keep in mind that there is no point in rushing through this exercise. You have to take your time and only move further down your body once you can feel that the part you have focused on is truly relaxed.

More importantly, I was told that if I did this exercise regularly, my brain would internalize it and I could eventually do it within a second or two.

This is exactly what happened.

After a few months, I was able to trigger off this exercise, which would take me all of a couple of seconds to complete, and then I would feel relaxed and revitalized. I began to use the exercise whenever I was feeling any stress at all, and eventually I habitualized even this aspect; now my brain triggers the exercise whenever it senses any stress, thus making sure that I don't reach a stressful state. (You may like to refer back to the earlier section on trigger points and habitualization, though in this case the habit is a positive one.)

Having said that, I am not immune when major, life-changing events occur. But I can honestly say that much of what I have done over the three decades or so since learning this technique, I could only do because I had learned how to avoid falling into the negative stress spiral.

Eliminating stress allows you to be more focused, to work faster and to make decisions more effectively. You start to not only embrace change but to love it, and you become happy to try new things without fear of failure.

Don't get me wrong – I've made my fair share of poor decisions, and with hindsight I can see plenty of opportunities I missed or wrong paths I have chosen, but I am nevertheless convinced that much of my success, such as it is, has been due to what I learned more than thirty years ago from Professor Parikh.

4 Eliminating stress-related headaches

There is just one more point I would like to add here: how to eliminate stress-related headaches from your life.

If you have a headache because you bumped your head, got wacked in a game of sport, taken medication that triggers headaches as a side effect, or – worst-case scenario – you have a brain tumor or other serious illness that affects your brain, then the following technique will not help you. The vast majority of headaches are, however, related to stress, and these are headaches you don't need to have.

Even headaches that come from drinking too much the night before often fall into the stress-headache category. Most likely (most of) the alcohol has been processed by your body. Dehydration may be a cause and you should drink plenty of water, but there is also likely a remaining sensitivity in your brain, which you can feel as a headache. As with stress, once you have a headache, you are more sensitive to the environment; even minor sensory experiences (such as a noise) can take your headache to a new level.

Your headache is simply an irritation that can take you on a downward spiral of sensitivity to even worse headaches. However, you can detach yourself from the headache, just as you learned to detach yourself from stress.

The simplest method is this:

Sit down, close your eyes and relax. Do a relaxation exercise.

Then focus on your headache and ask yourself the following questions:
- *How heavy is it?*
- *How big is it?*
- *What color is it?*

When you have answered these questions in your mind, do the relaxation exercise again. Then ask yourself the same questions again.

You will find that your headache will be lighter (maybe it has gone from feeling like 1 ton to 100 kg), smaller (maybe from 'filling my whole head' to 'about the size of a coin') and paler in color (perhaps from purple or black to light blue). Note that most people have to go through three or four rounds of this exercise before the headache disappears altogether.

Hopefully, you don't have headaches often, but if you suffer from headaches frequently, I recommend that you continue to use this technique consistently. After a while, you will find that you have established a trigger in your mind. As soon as you start the exercise, your headache starts to diminish and gradually vanishes.

Let me stress again, however, that this technique does not work if there are physical reasons for your headache, such as an illness or bumping your head. Having said that, I am yet to meet anyone who has tried this method for their stress-related headaches and found it not to work.

12

Food choices and exercise

You may find it strange that a book on weight loss doesn't focus on food and exercise.

There are reasons for keeping my focus on managing your mind rather than on what you eat or how physically active you are:

First, losing weight requires you to change your behavior and this book aims at helping you to become more effective in doing so. The principles of behavior change are the same regardless of whether you want to lose weight, to exercise more, stop smoking, become more productive, save more money, pass an exam or spend more time with your family.

Learning to address the key barriers to change that you are facing with respect to weight loss, will make you more effective when addressing other changes you want to make. Remember the willpower research quoted earlier? When you train your willpower by focusing on one particular challenge (such as weight loss) you will find that your willpower is also stronger when addressing other challenges (such as exercising more).

Second, there are plenty of books, magazine articles and on-line resources you can consult, should you want to learn more about food choices or exercise.

With respect to food there are massive cultural differences one needs to take into account. There is no point in presenting specific recipes or guidelines based on, say, an Anglo eating culture, when you happen to live in Thailand, India or China. In many countries there are extensive, credible, on-line sources that will help you make better food choices.

One of the best on-line resources is the US Food Pyramid, a program that has been updated and covers a wide range of topics. You might think that the web address is something like www.foodpyramid.com but it is not! You find it on www.cnpp.usda.gov. You will find dietary guidelines, information on lifecycle nutrition, diet and disease, food composition as well as a nutrition assistance program and surveys, reports and research.

Naturally, there is also a *weight and obesity* section, which again covers a wide range of topics. You can look up calories or nutrients in food, calculate your Body Mass Index, find healthy recipes, get practical, healthy weight control tips, or use the free weight tracker that is offered on-line. There are many more topics covered on that site. As already mentioned, if you live in a country with a vastly different food culture you can use the general guidelines offered by this website, but you will have to look for a local resource that offers you guidelines that are aligned with your country's food culture. I note that the US food pyramid site offers links to various ethnic food guidelines.

Whichever resources you use, the key to success is to follow the same *approach* I have proposed for your weight loss journey: Take a small step changing your food choices. Then allow yourself time to get used to the change and only when you are sure that you can maintain the change take the next small step.

Your focus needs to be on maintenance, i.e., on maintaining good habits. It will take time for you to make all the changes you want to make, but you will then be able to maintain them which, after all, is more important than impressive early successes followed by failure.

For most people the first step should be to add some healthy food to your diet (unless your diet is already healthy) as this will provide your body with more of the nutrients it needs. You should also decrease your food intake by starting to decrease your portion sizes and, over time, cutting out food you only eat because of bad habits or stress, such as snacks, additional courses when having a main meal or second (or third!) serves.

As the subtitle of this book states, it is about the neuroscience of weight loss. Learn to manage your mind and you will not only reach and maintain a Happy Weight, you will also be more effective in making whatever changes you want to make in your life.

13
Celebrate! Anything! Now!

An important rule of managing change is that you need to celebrate even small successes. The ability to celebrate is something that is unique to the human species, and it is likely that we have developed this capability for good reason.

Celebrations not only bring people closer together, they can also have a highly positive impact on an individual. But while it may be more fun to celebrate with others, it is something you should also consider doing on your own when you simply feel like it.

There is nothing wrong with celebrating success, but we should not limit ourselves to just that. It is important that we can be spontaneous and celebrate a nice day, sunshine, feeling good or even celebrate the fact that we are celebrating.

Limiting celebrations to particular achievements trains you to simply focus on these. Once that happens, you are likely to find that as soon as you have achieved something, you are already focusing on the next hurdle you intend to take, and your celebration becomes something of a routinized affair.

I am not suggesting that achievements don't deserve such

attention – they do. But they should be just one element in the mix of celebrations you engage in.

Having mentioned spontaneity, I should say a few more words about this quality.

For many people, life has become quite predictable. In fact, research undertaken in the USA shows that we do more or less the same things in the same places at around the same times for almost half of our lives.

For many people, meals, grocery shopping (and other regular shopping trips), working, personal hygiene (showering, brushing our teeth, etc.), driving to work, and so forth, all qualify as routine.

In a research study I found that quite a number of people even routinize their entertainment. For example, they may habitually have a barbecue and drink a certain brand of beer whenever they entertain one particular group of friends, but eat around the dining room table and drink a particular brand of wine with another group of friends.

As we have seen, routinization can be useful. For a start, you don't have to make decisions whenever you repeat an activity, which frees your brain up to engage with other possibly more interesting topics. But at the same time, you kill spontaneity and the spirit and energy that come with it. The popular saying 'being in a rut' suggests that it is a problem when life becomes too routinized.

Spontaneity often creates positive surprises, and surprises can enrich your life. Doing the same things the same way all the time is draining, while being surprised or exploring and discovering tend to be energizing. Doing the same things does not create new memories, while spontaneity is likely to do so. This means you will have more memories to draw on, enjoy, and refer to when making decisions, and you can utilize when trying to find creative solutions to a problem.

Most importantly, spontaneity is a means of giving you the feeling of having a greater degree of control over your life. The main problem with being in a rut is that people often feel trapped. They see themselves as being caught in routines, stuck in a predictable life that offers little but the same thing over and over. This naturally results in the feeling that one has little influence over one's present or future. A related problem is that too much routinized life robs you of the feeling that you are competent in dealing with different situations and challenges.

An extreme expression of this is the fact that many long-term prisoners feel inadequate returning to a normal life. They are so used to pre-determined routines that they find it hard to cope with the many decisions they have to make after they are released. Sadly, the incidence of re-incarceration and suicide within this population is quite high.

Obviously, living your life as though stuck in a rut is a long way from enforced prison routines, but it is nevertheless true that many people who have not done something different for a long time start to lose confidence in their ability to do so. When you have a highly varied life, you are likely to feel more competent in handling unexpected new situations and feel much more on top of things.

My final recommendation is this: celebrate right now! Maybe the sun is shining today, or you happen to find yourself in great company. Or simply celebrate that you have completed working through this book and have started to take charge...

A final word...

It may well be human nature to let the difficulties we face (rather than the good things we have and experience) determine how we feel about life. However, by doing so, we tend to get frustrated, anxious, angry, or just plain irritated. More often than not, this is just a massive waste of energy that exhausts us and saps our spirit.

The truth is, there is really no point in fretting about difficulties we can't avoid.

I am not suggesting that we shouldn't ever feel bad or even defeated, but that we should feel these for only long enough to digest what we are facing before moving on. Our challenge is to make friends of our unavoidable difficulties and then address the difficulties we *can* resolve. If we can't do this, we will find that the challenges we face will have a very significant negative impact on our life.

Looking at other cultures, we can see that elsewhere the idea of focusing on what we can change rather than what we can't is well entrenched. You may have heard of karma, which refers to the life situation we find ourselves in. Sometimes we have contributed to an unfavorable situation (and, hopefully, we have learned how to avoid that in future), but often we are just the victims of circumstance, and there is nothing we could have done to avoid the situation we find ourselves in. Our karma is that situation.

The recent global financial crisis and the subsequent European Sovereign Debt Crisis are a case in point. It had a devastating impact on many people. Some lost their homes, others their jobs, others again had to put their grand plans for the future on hold. Many people experienced profound anxiety when thinking about their future.

There was, of course, nothing they could do about the recession. Naturally, they felt upset, frustrated, anxious, angry – especially because they couldn't do anything to make the pressures caused by the recession go away.

But what can all this frustration, anger and anxiety contribute? Certainly it cannot provide a solution to their problems. What they get, instead, is a life made even more miserable because of the negative energy generated by focusing on these difficulties.

The challenge is to snap out of feeling like a helpless victim and, instead, to work within the more limited territory where positive actions can be taken.

While we can't change karma – the situation we find ourselves in – we still have choices we can make in the way we deal with our situation. This is called dharma. Karma is the hand we have been dealt in this round of the great poker game of life, while dharma is how we play the cards we have been dealt, regardless of how good a hand it is.

Karma is a given, and negative energy expended on it is wasted energy. Dharma, on the other hand, can be shaped by our decisions. Our challenge is to deal with our karma in an effective way and not to waste our energy stewing in negative feelings or feeling sorry for ourselves because of our 'bad' karma.

How we use the time, skills and resources we have under our command – regardless of how diminished these may be – is key to making progress. Rather than decry what we have lost or cannot have, we need to focus on what we can do in the situation we are in. Maybe we can learn new skills or advance a hobby, because we finally have time to do so. Perhaps we can reduce stress and pressure and give our body and mind a break.

You may well accuse me of being superficial and flippant, having not experienced your own situation first hand. You are right to do so. But let me tell you a true story:

Viktor Frankl was a leading psychologist living in Vienna during World War II. Being Jewish, he was dragged off to a concentration camp. He survived the camp, and in his book *Man's Search for Meaning,* he tells of physically strong men who did not survive because they simply could not see anything worth living for, while weaker men (and he himself was not particularly physically strong) survived because they still saw meaning in their life, despite their karma.

He believed that many people suffer from not being able to

find meaning in the life they live. They are unable to accept their karma, and this keeps them from moving forward in their life. Frankl developed Logotherapy (*Logos* is 'meaning' in Greek), and the insights he gained during a phase of his life that was worse than any experience the vast majority of people will ever have to endure were spot on.

We need to make a superhuman effort never to get lost in bad karma. Naturally, we will need some time to adjust and digest, but then we need to move on as soon as we can and focus on dharma, i.e., what we can constructively do despite the situation we find ourselves in. If we don't do this, we will find that the negative energy we generate by focusing on a situation we can't change will poison our life, sap our energy, and limit our ability to move forward.

This needs to be avoided at all costs.

Whatever it is that we *can* do needs to be the focus of our attention, rather than what we can't change. In fact, the sooner we get at a healthy emotional distance from any bad karma, the sooner we can start to enjoy whatever opportunities – large or small – are still open to us.

Part of this positive approach to life is to change what we don't like about the way we live when the only thing holding us back from making such a change is ourselves: bad habits, an unwillingness to take risks, a lack of happiness despite what we have already achieved in our life, an inability to deal with – or even eliminate – stress, a fear of failure, or an inability to enjoy what works well for us, even if it is not perfect.

My objective with the Happy Weight book is to highlight how you can break down some of the barriers that hold you back.

But this publication is not about recipes but rather about starting points. It is not about telling you what to do, but about explaining what is happening to you – and to millions of other people who find it difficult to reach and maintain their Happy Weight. I have achieved my goal if I have provided you with useful insights and starting points and convinced you that you *can* take charge.

There is no such thing as a single strategy that works for everyone. As long as you take charge, experiment, explore, learn more about what does and doesn't work for you, and develop, you are making progress, and I have no doubt you will eventually reach and maintain your Happy Weight!

Send me an email if you have any questions or comments or simply want to be kept informed about future Happy Weight publications or activities.
*My email address is **peter@petersteidl.com***

Appendix

11 insights that help you understand your mind

It should be clear by now that we have to deal with the way our mind works if we want to change our behavior, regardless of what sort of change that might be. The more we understand about how our mind works, the more likely are we to develop effective ways of making the changes we want to make.

In this Appendix I present 11 insights that will help you understand your mind better. If you are not interested don't read through them: this section is for the curious. It is not necessary for you to delve that far into this subject matter to successfully lose weight. Personally I feel that knowing more about how our mind works can only help - if not with your weight loss challenge then with other aspects of your life you want to change...

Insight 1: You think in images and emotions

Here is a brief exercise:

Close your eyes and think about what you had for breakfast.

What came to your mind? Words that described the food that you ate? Or pictures of what you had? If words came up in your mind, you should see someone about it – that's not good at all! But most likely you would have seen an image.

I could just as well have asked you to think about something really good that happened in your life, or something really bad. You would find that after a few minutes you start feeling good (or, in the latter case, bad).

This happens because your brain, unlike a computer, stores not only information but also *feelings*. These sensations and emotional reactions are very powerful, and they are recalled just like other memories. This is why you may start to feel angry or tense when you think about a particularly bad experience in your past. You don't just recall the information, but you recall and therefore feel the emotions associated with that experience.

It follows that when you get upset while waiting in a queue at the checkout, you are not only likely to recall other occasions when you had to wait for a long time, but also the negative feelings, such as frustration and anger, that compound the negativity of your current situation. Let me add one more exercise:

Think back to a novel you have read and greatly enjoyed and a novel you did not enjoy at all.

Would it be right to say that, for the novel you enjoyed, you could actually 'see' the characters and what was happening in your mind while you were reading the novel, while in the latter case you didn't?

I am sure you have come across the argument that stories are powerful, or you may have come to that conclusion based on your own experience. This is, of course, only half the story: stories are powerful when they allow the listener or reader to *see* the story and feel the emotions. Even better, when they see themselves in this story.

But stories are not at all effective when they are simply received as a sequence of words that don't activate any emotional involvement.

Conclusion: Images and emotions are the language of the mind. We have to use images and emotions to reach and influence our non-conscious mind.

Insight 2: You can experience what other people experience by observing them

Mirror neurons allow us to experience the feelings of others. They are highly effective and can flood your whole brain with strong feelings when you see another person in a high-emotion situation.

Here is an exercise:

Think of a movie, a play, an awards ceremony, or a news item that triggered emotions in you. You may have felt frightened when a character in a thriller walked into a trap, or felt teary when a family or relationship situation was resolved with high emotion.

Think about these occasions: Were you able to feel the emotions these other people must have felt? Why did YOU feel these emotions?

Our mirror neurons allow us to feel what others feel without actually being in their place. It follows that we can allow somebody to experience benefits or, alternatively, problems by showing them how other people experience them.

But to do that, we need to create a high-emotion situation. Mirror neurons can't be activated by rationality. Being told that somebody really enjoyed the benefits of, say, losing weight doesn't work. We need to expose the person to the positive emotions the person who has lost weight has experienced.

Conclusion: We can help the mind experience emotions by showing other people in highly emotional situations.

Insight 3: Your emotions are driving your decisions

We know that this is the case: accident victims who have

damaged the emotional centre of the brain can have a perfectly normal discussion with you. But they can't make even the simplest decision.

All decisions require emotions - however, this does not mean that you are necessarily aware of the specific emotions involved in a decision you make.

Emotions are designed to help us adapt to the environment and to survive. When the brain stores past experiences in memory it also stores associated emotions. When making a decision, high emotion memories are given more weight than low emotion memories.

Emotions determine what matters to us and which of the millions of signals that reach our mind we are becoming aware of. Emotions tell us what is important to be remembered, help us recall memories and guide our decisions. The more richly an event is categorized by emotion, the longer and more detailed it will be remembered.

Conclusion: We cannot tell our non-conscious mind to do things. But we can use emotions to get it to do something.

Insight 4: How you see the world today is based on what you experienced in the past

I am not talking about some traumatic experience that can mark somebody for life, but rather about the simple, typically quite uneventful, day-to-day life most of us live.

Let's start with a simple exercise:

Close your eyes for a minute and think about Coca Cola.[14]

You may have seen the Coke can or bottle in your mind, the logo, perhaps the beach or a picnic table, you may have recalled the taste of Coke or an occasion when you drank it.

Whatever it was that flooded into your mind is obviously something you have been exposed to in the past.

And these past memories determine the way you feel about Coca Cola, and the likelihood of you choosing to drink Coke in the future or recommending or serving it to others.

The way you see your world is based on the memories you have collected over time.

You also know from your own experience that when you haven't 'used' memories - when you haven't thought of something for a long time - they slowly fade. You forget...

What happens is that the connections between neurons that carry these memories get weaker and weaker until the memory has faded away. The memory is actually still in your mind, but you are no longer able to access it.

This means that it is partly *what* you have experienced, and partly *how often* you have thought about these experiences, that

---

[14] If you have no memory of Coca Cola try Pepsi, Red Bull, McDonalds or a product or place you know well.

will determine how you see the world.

Conclusion: If we want our mind to see the world differently, we have to create new experiences that become memories.

Insight 5: You brain creates stronger memories for negative experiences

Our brain is designed to create stronger memories of negative experiences than for positive ones.

This of course makes sense when living in a hostile environment, as learning from and remembering threats and tricky situations is essential for survival, while having enjoyable memories is nice, but not essential.

In today's world, however, this means that we all too easily feel guilty, less than confident or unable to cope, simply because negative experiences are imprinted so much more strongly than positive ones.

Conclusion: We have to take great care to balance negative experiences with lots of positive ones, because the positive will create much weaker memories than the negative. And, remember, these memories determine how you see your world!

Insight 6: 'You' don't decide what to 'put into memory' – your non-conscious mind decides...

Here is another exercise:

Close your eyes (without first trying to remember what you see).

Then, with your eyes closed, try to remember all the details of the room you are in or, if you are not alone in this room, try to recall the details of other people – their clothes (fabric, color, style), accessories, personal features (eye, hair and skin color, facial features, body features), and so forth.

After a couple of minutes open your eyes again and see what you have missed. Most likely you were not able to recall much detail at all.

Does this mean that your senses didn't transmit all the details to your brain? You don't need to worry; your senses are automatically transmitting even the finest details. But your mind places only a small selection of these into your memory.

In fact, your brain uses a chemical process that eliminates all signals that it deems to be of little relevance to you. You are not even aware of this process that takes place in your brain all the time.

So it should not come as a surprise that some 95+ per cent of your thinking happens in the non-conscious. It happens, but you are not aware of what is happening.

Conclusion: If we want to create new or change existing memories we have to create *memorable* experiences. Memorable experiences are those that are about ourselves, are strongly emotional, surprising, or link into memories we already have.

Insight 7: Your mind links memories

Let's start with an exercise:

Have you had experiences similar to these?

- *A particular smell reminds you of a holiday or of your childhood. As soon as this happens, images related to this particular event or situation start to surface in your mind, and you remember fragments or even large parts of these experiences.*

- *You taste something that reminds you of another eating occasion, leading to memories of where you were or with whom you had that meal.*

- *You are waiting for service in a long queue and suddenly you recall other situations where you had to wait for a long time before being served, and how frustrated you were.*

You are *not* consciously trying to remember all this. But when one part of the memory is activated by an experience or thought, your mind automatically activates other, connected memory units.

Parts of the same memory are stored in different parts of the brain, creating a number of linked neural networks. When you remember something, your brain reconstitutes the memory by piecing the bits of the puzzle together.

This also means that every time you call up a memory you change it. You may not call up all of the neuronal networks that carry related content because some connections may have become weak.

At the same time, you may have connected new content with parts of a memory that *is* called up, and this will impact on what you seem to remember.

Essentially, we can say with certainty that none of our memories are totally accurate. Some are likely to have been distorted much more than others, but any memory that is called up will change...

Conclusion: We need to associate anything we want the non-conscious mind to commit to with a positive experience. For example, we can celebrate small steps forward as a way of linking a positive experience (the celebration) to achieving the change in behavior we are trying to make.

Insight 8: Your expectations have a significant impact on your experience

What is or isn't a great experience depends very much on how a particular experience stacks up against an individual's past experiences.

For example, black & white television offered a most desirable, fantastic experience when it was launched, but today

– because we're used to color television – it would have little if any appeal. Similarly, what young people used to find exciting a generation ago is very different to what today's young people find exciting, because today's youth have been – and continue to be – exposed to much more dynamic experiences.

The same principle applies to day-to-day exposures and the development of expectations. When you can withdraw money from an ATM within seconds, you find waiting in a bank branch more annoying than you ever did. However, if you are used to banks in some developing countries where it takes you several hours to conclude a simple transaction, you may find a ten minute wait in your home bank a highly positive experience.

Clearly, new experiences can lead to a 're-classification' of old memories and, by doing so, can also change the impact future experiences will have.

Think about the following:

Can you think of examples where past experiences raised expectations with respect to future experiences, like going back to a place you liked, or catching up with a person you used to have a great time with, and expecting a similarly positive experience? This would confirm that past experiences have an impact on your expectations.

Conclusion: Be aware of your expectations. You will enjoy life more when your expectations are not unrealistic.

Insight 9: You can prime your mind

A specific aspect of managing expectations is *priming*.

Priming is a process that raises certain expectations and, by doing so, changes the way subsequent experiences are interpreted.

For example, taking a headache tablet is likely to lead to the headache subsiding well before the medication could possibly have had a physiological effect. The brain, being aware that a tablet has been taken and expecting that this tablet will have an impact, starts to reduce the pain level even before the medication starts to work.

There are also the classic 'taste tests' where a third rate drink (such as wine) is poured from a bottle showing a leading brand. Invariably, many people are primed by the label and expect a superior taste experience. And because of this expectation, they rate the taste much more favorably than they rate the same drink when it is served from a bottle carrying a label from an inferior brand.

We also know from fMRI studies (i.e., using advanced medical diagnostic technology) that our brain processes a drink we *expect* to be superior differently to one we expect to be inferior.

Conclusion: It is as important to manage expectations as it is to manage the eventual experience.

Insight 10: You can experience emotions through visualization

Visualization allows us to reach our non-conscious, to create emotions, activate (if we want) mirror neurons, develop new memories, and prime the non-conscious mind.

Imagine you are pursuing a long-term goal that requires you to change your behavior today, as a first and early step towards realizing this goal. This means that you won't experience the benefits for some time, but you need to get your non-conscious mind on board today.

We already know that our non-conscious 'old brain' doesn't understand logic and reason. To get our non-conscious brain on board we need to allow it to experience emotional benefits and, given that these benefits are not yet real, we have to imagine them.

This may sound a bit weird but is, in fact, a practice widely used in sports psychology.

In sports psychology, the focus is on imagining the emotional rewards of winning. In your case it is a matter of imagining the emotional rewards of succeeding, i.e., making the change you want to make, and sustaining your new behavior.

It is important that you don't just imagine the actual outcome, but rather the positive emotions you will feel when you achieve that outcome. These are the rewards your old brain is seeking and will experience as a result of the changes you are planning to make.

Ideally, these rewards should be embellished as much as possible – you should go into great detail imagining how you will feel telling a friend about your new job or how they will admire you for having lost weight or given up smoking (or whatever it is that you are working towards); how you will feel when you are finally free of a burden; how you will feel on top of your life when you've taken charge of your own destiny; and so forth.

If you find all this a bit airy-fairy, consider that your imagination can trigger the same processes in your brain that take place when you experience the 'real thing'.

For example, experiments have shown that people who imagine physical exercise don't boost their muscle strength as much as people who actually undertake these exercises, but they do build muscle strength nevertheless.

You probably also know from your own experience that imagining something really sad makes you feel sad, while imagining something positive and happy lifts your spirits. In these and other cases the brain is tricked into releasing the same chemicals it would normally release in a real world situation. Once those chemicals are released, the impact is much the same, whether the situation is real or imaginary.

Conclusion: Visualization is a highly effective way to 'talk' to your non-conscious mind and to let it experience future emotional rewards today.

Insight 11: Your mind responds to the demands you make on it

I don't know you, but I do know something about you – I know that you are smarter than your grandparents were.

How do I know that?

Dr Flynn, a New Zealand University Professor, analyzed IQ scores for up to 80 years back covering some 14 countries. And there was one consistent feature that stood out: his analyses showed that, across all countries and at all times, there was clear evidence that every generation is smarter than the previous one.

So there is a very good chance that your are smarter than your parents, who are smarter than your grandparents, who are smarter than your great-grandparents, and so forth. It is also very likely that your children are smarter than you.

But why are we all getting smarter?

The reason is that our brain adapts to the demands we make on it. Today's children play more demanding games, live in an environment that is more complex than the one we grew up in, and are encouraged - if not forced - to learn things we had never heard about when we were their age.

And dealing with this ever-increasing complexity and challenge pushes the brain to allocate additional neurons to the task allowing it to do more and better, which results in an increase in intelligence scores.

Let me give you another example that shows how the brain adapts to demands:

A study of London taxi drivers showed that the part of their brain that deals with spatial challenges - like imagining a map in your mind to work out how to best get from A to B - is significantly larger than for the average person. The taxi drivers' brains have allocated more neurons to this task, simply because they regularly use their brain to work out which way to take passengers to their destination.

Conclusion: You can 'train your brain'.

About the Author

Dr Peter Steidl has lived in Austria, Germany, the United Kingdom and Australia and has carried out assignments in 20 countries on five continents. He has an MBA and PhD from Vienna University.

But it has been his work rather than his studies that have allowed him to gain insights into how people think, what they fear, and how they make decisions.

Over the years he met with more than 20,000 people face-to-face in small discussion groups and in-depth interviews. He has spent time with home makers, students, unemployed people, professionals, entrepreneurs, unskilled workers, volunteers, managers, executives and board members; young and old people; people in developed and developing countries; men and women.

Always interested in new experiences, he has been a Temporary Advisor to the World Health Organization, represented Australia at the European Center for Social Science Research and Documentation, represented Austria as Honorary Consul for South Australia and the Northern Territory, and served on government boards and committees as well as on the boards of not-for-profit organizations.

Having been exposed to different cultures, people, situations and experiences, he realized that at the end of the day the vast majority of people struggle with the very same issues. Importantly, these issues are typically created by what we call progress - progress that has created a world that is very different to the one humans lived in for millions of years.

This rapid change in the environment, in the challenges we face, and the goals we set ourselves is creating problems because our brains are not designed to deal with them. Our brains have been fine-tuned over millions of years to survive in, and adapt to, a hostile physical environment, and much unhappiness, frustration, resignation and even ill-health stems from the dissonance between the way our brain works and the challenges we face in today's world.

This book represents an attempt to explain why it is so difficult for so many people, who are clearly intelligent and committed, to lose weight, and to provide practical steps than can be taken to move towards a more satisfying and happier life by reaching and maintaining your Happy Weight.

Peter values any feedback or comments you are willing to provide. He can be contacted at **peter@petersteidl.com**

References

Ariely, Dan	*Predictable Irrationality: The Hidden Forces that Shape Our Decisions*, London 2009
Burka, Jane B & Lenora M Yuen	*Procrastination: Why You Do It, What to Do about Now*, Cambridge 2008
Doidge, Norman	*The Brain that Changes Itself*, New York 2007
Duggan, William	*Strategic Intuition: The Creative Spark in Human Achievement*, New York 2007
Duhigg, Charles	*The Power of Habit. Why We Do What We Do in Life and Business*, New York 2012
Earls, Mark	*Herd: How to Change Mass Behaviour by Harnessing Our True Nature*, West Sussex 2009
Frankl, Viktor E.	*Man's Search for Meaning*, New York 1984
Gardner, Howard	*Intelligence Reframed: Multiple Intelligences for the 21st Century*, New York 2002

Gardner, Howard   *Changing Minds: The Arts and Science of Changing Our Own and Other People's Minds*, Boston 2004

Hammond, Claudia   *Emotional Rollercoaster: A Journey through the Science of Feelings*, London 2006

Johnson, Steven   *Everything Bad is Good for You*, London 2006

Keen, Andrew   *The Cult of the Amateur: How Today's Internet is Killing Our Culture and Assaulting Our Economy*, London 2007

Klein, Gary   *The Power of Intuition*, New York 2003

Klein, Gary   *Streetlights and Shadows: Searching for the Keys to Adaptive Decision Making*, Cambridge 2009

Lawrence, Paul R. and Nitin Nohria   *Driven: How Human Nature Shapes Our Choices*, San Francisco 2002

Martin, Neale   *Habit: The 95% of Behavior Marketers Ignore*, New Jersey 2008

McGonigal, Kelly   *The Willpower Instinct: How Self-Control Works, Why It Matters, and What You Can Do to Get More of It*, New York 2012

Mlodinow, Leonard — *Subliminal. How your unconscious mind rules your behavior*, New York 2012

Parikh, Jagdish — *Managing Your Self: Management by Detached Involvement*, Oxford 1991

Pink, Daniel H. — *A Whole New Mind: Moving from the Information Age to the Conceptual Age*, New York 2005

Pink, Daniel H. — *Drive: The Surprising truth about what motivates us*, New York 2009

Pinker, Steven — *The Blank Slate*, London 2002

Schwartz, Barry — *The Paradox of Choice: Why More is Less. How the Culture of Abundance Robs Us of Satisfaction*, New York 2004

Strauch, Barbara — *The Secret Life of the Grown-up Brain*, New York 2010

Underwood, Geoffrey — *Oxford Guide to the Mind: Understand the Everyday Mysteries of the Human Mind*, Oxford 2001

Watson, Richard — *Future Minds: How the Digital Age is Changing Our Minds, Why This Matters and What We Can Do About It*, London 2010

Wilson, Timothy D.   *Strangers to Ourselves: Discovering the Adaptive Unconscious*, Cambridge 2002

Wilson, Timothy D.   *Redirect: The surprising new science of psychological change*, New York 2011

Winston, Robert   *The Human Mind and How to Make the Most of It*, London 2003